Joanie Greggains'
Total Shape-up

Joanie Greggains' Total

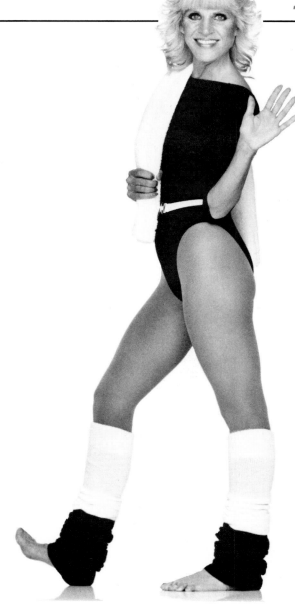

Shape-up

by Joanie Greggains
with John Foreman

Photographs by John Jensen

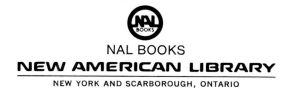

NAL BOOKS
NEW AMERICAN LIBRARY
NEW YORK AND SCARBOROUGH, ONTARIO

Copyright © 1984 by Joanie Greggains
All rights reserved. For information address New American Library
Published simultaneously in Canada by
The New American Library of Canada Limited

NAL BOOKS TRADEMARK REG. U.S. PAT. OFF. AND FOREIGN COUNTRIES
REGISTERED TRADEMARK—MARCA REGISTRADA
HECHO EN CRAWFORDSVILLE, INDIANA, U.S.A.

SIGNET, SIGNET CLASSIC, MENTOR, PLUME, MERIDIAN and
NAL BOOKS are published *in the United States* by New American
Library, 1633 Broadway, New York, New York 10019, *in Canada* by
The New American Library of Canada Limited, 81 Mack Avenue,
Scarborough, Ontario M1L 1M8

LIBRARY OF CONGRESS CATALOGING IN PUBLICATION DATA
Greggains, Joanie.
Joanie Greggains' Total shape-up.
Includes index.
1. Reducing exercises.   2. Exercise for women.
3. Reducing diets.   4. Vegetarian cookery. I. Foreman,
John, 1945-   .   II. Title.
RA781.6.G74   1984   613.7′1   83-25448
ISBN 0-453-00455-5

Designed by Kathryn Parise

First Printing, May, 1984

1 2 3 4 5 6 7 8 9

PRINTED IN THE UNITED STATES OF AMERICA

Contents

Introduction

Hi Fitness Fans!

Now I've gone and written my very own book—with the help of my dazzlingly handsome co-author, of course. In it is everything I've ever thought should be in a fitness book.

I put a lot of work into it to give you my special brand of totally energizing exercises that utilize many, many muscles instead of only a few.

Exercise, as we all know, makes us look good and feel good too. An unbeatable combination. The Total Shape-up plan is really easy to use. You'll love it. You'll love the diet too.

Just remember, there's nothing that your little body can't do *as long as* 1) you work up to it at your own pace, and 2) you don't give up!

Have fun shaping up, and send me a copy of your chart when you're done!

Let's go!

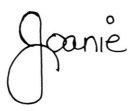

Joanie Greggains'
Total Shape-up

The Total Shape-up— How It Works

Maybe recently you haven't done anything more strenuous than tear open packages of Twinkies and switch television channels.

Maybe you're one of those who avoid exercise out of embarrassment. "Go to a pool? I'd be harpooned!"

Or maybe you're a sleek professional looking for a terrific new way to work out.

Whoever you are, here's a program you can do in private and with great results: the Total Shape-up.

Mondays, Wednesdays, and *Fridays* you work on *aerobics.* That's for the heart, your body's engine of energy.

Tuesdays and *Thursdays* you work on *toning* individual muscle groups. That's for physical beauty.

Don't worry. You'll never be bored. I've designed *three separate Total Shape-up cycles.* Each is meant to be used for three months, 30–40 minutes each day. At the end of the first three-month period of doing Total Shape-up I, switch to Total Shape-up II. After three more months, move on to Total Shape-up III. After nine full months, go back to Total Shape-up I, and cycle through again.

Each Total Shape-up is equally demanding; none is harder than the others. Your improving level of fitness will be reflected by the increased number of repetitions you can do in each, whether you're a modest novice or a pro.

Besides giving you variety, this rotation will enable you to work your muscles in slightly different ways. I think you'll find that this subtle change of emphasis every three months has a better over-all toning effect, and you will never be required to manage some limb-twisting, excessively aerobic extravaganza labeled "advanced."

Aerobics

Simple definition: any exercise or activity that elevates the heart rate to *at least* 120 beats per minute for *at least* 12 minutes is said to be aerobic.

So what does this mean? Well, the heartbeat keeps us alive, and the *only* way to condition the heart is through aerobics. Remember that your heart is a muscle. It can't do little push-ups or lift little weights. If it's to get any exercise you've got to do something that gets you huffing and puffing and sweating. Otherwise your heart won't pound. And if it never pounds, it'll do what any unexercised muscle does—get flabby. Flabby hearts work harder to pump the same amount of blood through your system. And they make everything you do—from getting out of bed to reaching over to tie your shoe—a little tougher.

The only way to really nurture your natural store of vitality and energy is by *conditioning your heart.* If it's firm and fit you'll feel great. If it's limp and spongy you won't. Diet control is critical to good health and good looks, but don't put the cart before the horse. For energy you need aerobics.

The key to measuring your aerobic progress is knowing how to measure your heart rate. There are four rates you'll need to determine.

The first is your *resting heartbeat.* This is just the average number of beats per minute when you're not doing any strenuous activity. Most people have resting heart rates somewhere between 65 and 85 beats per minute. Athletes in the peak of condition are down around 39 beats per minute. If you subscribe to the theory that life span is a finite number of heartbeats then you'll agree that the lower your heart rate the better. Even if you don't hold with this theory, common sense would suggest that a heart beating all day at a rate of 85 is likely to wear out earlier than one doing the same work but at a rate of 60. In fact, it's an accepted medical fact that lowering the resting heart rate is good for the health. And a low resting heart rate is also the true test of fitness.

The best time to measure your resting heart rate is in the morning when you first wake up, before caffeine. Put the fingers of one hand on the carotid artery on the side of your neck. You have two carotids, so take your pick. You'll feel it pulsing in time with your heart as it runs between the collarbone and the jawline midway between the Adam's apple and each side of the neck. With the other hand, take a watch with a sweep second hand and see how many beats you count in a 10-second interval. You must be calm and undisturbed. Multiply the number of beats in the 10-second interval by six and the result will closely approximate your resting heart rate. Average is 72 for men, 80 for women, 50 for athletes of either sex. Anything under 40 is marathon material.

Now we come to *maximum heart rate.* This is a danger line beyond which you should never push yourself. You determine your maximum heart rate by subtracting your age from a constant 220. For example, if you are 40 years old, subtracting 40 from 220 will yield a maximum heart rate of 180. The point of aerobics is to elevate the heart rate, but never as high as this.

It is the *target heart rate* that tells you exactly how hard you must work in order to condition your heart. This is the heart rate you want during and immediately after each workout. You calculate your target heart rate by multiplying the maximum heart rate by one of three constants: If you exercise regularly, multiply your maximum rate by .75; if you don't exercise but lead an active life, then multiply your maximum rate by .70; and finally if you smoke more than four cigarettes a day or are 20 pounds overweight or are recovering from a serious illness, then multiply your maximum rate by .65. One or another of these constants will yield the optimum number of heartbeats per minute during a workout.

Finally, there's the *working heart rate.* You calculate this pretty much as you did the resting rate. Except this time you count the beats in a 10-second period *immediately after* the aerobic workout. Multiply by six and that's your working heart rate. If it's at or above the level of your maximum heart rate, you're trying too hard. Go slower. If it's hardly above your resting rate, then you aren't trying hard enough. The closer it is to the target heart rate the better the conditioning effect on the heart.

There are places to note all these heart rates on your Progress Chart on page 7. Be sure you record each one and continue to do so as your exercise program continues.

Vital as aerobic exercise is, it doesn't work on the entire body. You need toning for your waist, stomach, arms and pectorals, thighs, hips, and bottom, in that order.

There are four purposes to these exercises. They will increase your muscles' *strength* so that you'll be able to do a greater range of activities; they will improve your muscles' *tone* so that they won't sag like drapes; they will increase your *flexibility;* and they will heighten your *endurance* so that you can finish things you used to be afraid to even start.

These are not spot reducing exercises. That's because *there's no such thing as spot reducing.* If you want to lose weight, you have to stop overeating and become active. There is no magic way to remove *just* the French bread over the bra, *just* the hanging armpits, *just* the cottage cheese on the thighs, or any of the other things men will never know about. And guys, that spare tire around the middle or the twin pontoons on your butt won't disappear either unless you tackle the *whole body.*

Only through total exercise will you use up enough energy to make a noticeable dent in that stored fat. Exercise burns calories, it's true. But the stored calories contained in fat burn a lot more slowly than you think. They also don't always come off in the places you want them to.

Alternately contracting and extending the muscles burns subcutaneous fat. But more important, it makes the muscles firm. That's something dieting alone can't do. Have you ever seen a compulsive eater who's skinny but also kind of flabby? It can happen when you just cut calories and don't do any exercise. And if it does happen, it defeats a major purpose of dieting, which is to look good. Flab looks bad. But it's what you wind up with—diet or no diet—if you lack good muscle tone.

The toning routines in this book aren't just exercises, they're patterns. Each movement builds toward the next. This is what makes the routines so much more effective than separate, nonrelated exercises. The rhythmic, constant, flowing motion you'll achieve has an aerobic effect as well as a toning effect. And because the toning exercises form patterns, they'll help your coordination and give you a feeling of control.

I've been a fitness professional for 15 years and can recognize boring exercises when I see them. Mine aren't. I've purposely made them like choreography instead of like boot camp. They'll make the whole process of exercising more enjoyable.

An exercise mat, or a big towel laid on the carpet, or anything to cushion the hard floor.

Tennis shoes or running shoes. No bare feet on aerobic days.

Comfortable clothes, like leotards. Don't wear anything tight or binding. And ladies, it's *much* more comfortable to wear a bra.

Clock or watch with a sweep second hand so that you can time your routines and accurately monitor your heart rate.

Music you love—fast tempo for warm-ups and aerobics, moderate tempo for toning exercises and cool-downs. Note: Records are better than tapes, simply because it's easy to move the needle around.

A book prop and rubber bands to keep this book open and in front of you until you learn the routines. A music stand is great, but no doubt you can improvise something else if you must.

An open window; it's hot doing exercises and there's nothing like fresh air when you're breathing hard.

A glass of water, from which you should sip occasionally during your workout.

Look for the notes on health when you're doing the routines, so that you can learn something about everything from laser face lifts to cellulite, from quick ways to get rid of a side stitch to a common supermarket item that increases the thickness of your hair!

To get the most from your Total Shape-up you'll want to modify your eating habits. I think that diet is so important that I've included an entire section on it at the end of the book, complete with my basic principles of good eating and recipes that are delicious as well as nutritious and low in calories. So be sure to make this diet part of your Total Shape-up!

• *Think positively.* Do you chronically belittle your body and appearance even in your inner thoughts? Then stop. Concentrate on the possibility of progress. Visualize your body the way you want it and work toward that goal. Do it consciously, and do it every day.

• *Find your prime time.* Some people like exercising in the morning, others prefer the afternoon, and still others have jobs or families that permit only certain in-between times alone. Decide on your prime time (or only time) and let it be known that you are *not* to be disturbed. Carve this time out of your schedule and make it sacred.

• *Give yourself time.* Don't squash exercises into a skimpy time slot between pressing or worrisome duties. Don't rush. Don't despair after a few weeks or months because you haven't metamorphosed into a butterfly. Remember, you gave yourself a great deal of time to overeat, lie around, and feel guilty. You can certainly afford the time to become fit and beautiful. Be patient and keep at it.

• *Don't overdo it.* Can't keep moving through the whole aerobic section? Fine; do what you can and rest when you have to. Can't touch your toes or bend your seated body all the way forward to the floor? Or twist the side of your thigh toward the ceiling? Again, no big deal. *I'm serious.* Do what you can and rest when you must. If you keep at this long enough eventually you'll be able to do *every single movement* as well as any pro. Just don't expect to be a pro right away. Even if a certain movement seems hopelessly impossible, *do the best you can.* Trying is better than nothing at all.

• *Reward yourself.* Not with a banana split, please. But at the end of three months when you're ready to move on to Total Shape-up II, take yourself out to a movie. Or buy a piece of attractive clothing whose purpose isn't to obscure the body. Or spring for a really nice leotard. Make the end of each Total Shape-up cycle an occasion for a little celebration of your progress and determination. Give yourself a present.

There is probably no other single thing that holds as much potential for future encouragement as a chart clearly demonstrating physical improvement. You're probably going to need this encouragement in the months to come. So by all means use your Progress Chart from the very start.

Chart Your Progress

PROGRESS CHART

AEROBIC

Target heart rate   _____beats/min.
Maximum heart rate   _____beats/min.

	Date (at start): _____	Date (at 3 months): _____	Date (at 6 months): _____	Date (at 1 year): _____
Working heart rate	_____beats/min.	_____beats/min.	_____beats/min.	_____beats/min.
Resting heart rate	_____beats/min.	_____beats/min.	_____beats/min.	_____beats/min.

TONING (The first week of each Total Shape-up cycle, just *learn* the routines. *Then* at the end of that week, note the total number of *repetitions* you can do of each routine.)

First Time Through:

	Total Shape-up I — Repetitions		Total Shape-up II — Repetitions		Total Shape-up III — Repetitions	
	Date (1 week after start):	Date (at 3 months):	Date (1 week after start):	Date (at 3 months):	Date (1 week after start):	Date (at 3 months):
Waist	____	____	____	____	____	____
Stomach	____	____	____	____	____	____
Arms and pectorals	____	____	____	____	____	____
Thighs	____	____	____	____	____	____
Hips	____	____	____	____	____	____
Bottom	____	____	____	____	____	____

Second Time Through:

	Total Shape-up I — Repetitions		Total Shape-up II — Repetitions		Total Shape-up III — Repetitions	
	Date (1 week after start):	Date (at 3 months):	Date (1 week after start):	Date (at 3 months):	Date (1 week after start):	Date (at 3 months):
Waist	____	____	____	____	____	____
Stomach	____	____	____	____	____	____
Arms and pectorals	____	____	____	____	____	____
Thighs	____	____	____	____	____	____
Hips	____	____	____	____	____	____
Bottom	____	____	____	____	____	____

In addition to keeping track of your physical progress on your Progress Chart, it'll be an extra boost to be able to see how much slimmer and trimmer you're getting!

Take Your
Measurements

MEASUREMENT CHART

	Start Date:_____	3 months Date:_____	6 months Date:_____	1 year Date:_____
Chest/bust	_____ in.	_____ in.	_____ in.	_____ in.
Upper arm	_____ in.	_____ in.	_____ in.	_____ in.
Waist	_____ in.	_____ in.	_____ in.	_____ in.
Hip	_____ in.	_____ in.	_____ in.	_____ in.
Upper thigh	_____ in.	_____ in.	_____ in.	_____ in.
Calf	_____ in.	_____ in.	_____ in.	_____ in.
Weight	_____ lbs.	_____ lbs.	_____ lbs.	_____ lbs.

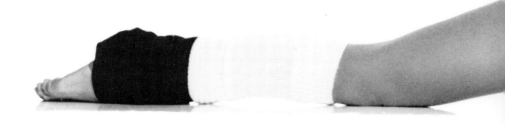

Total Shape-up I

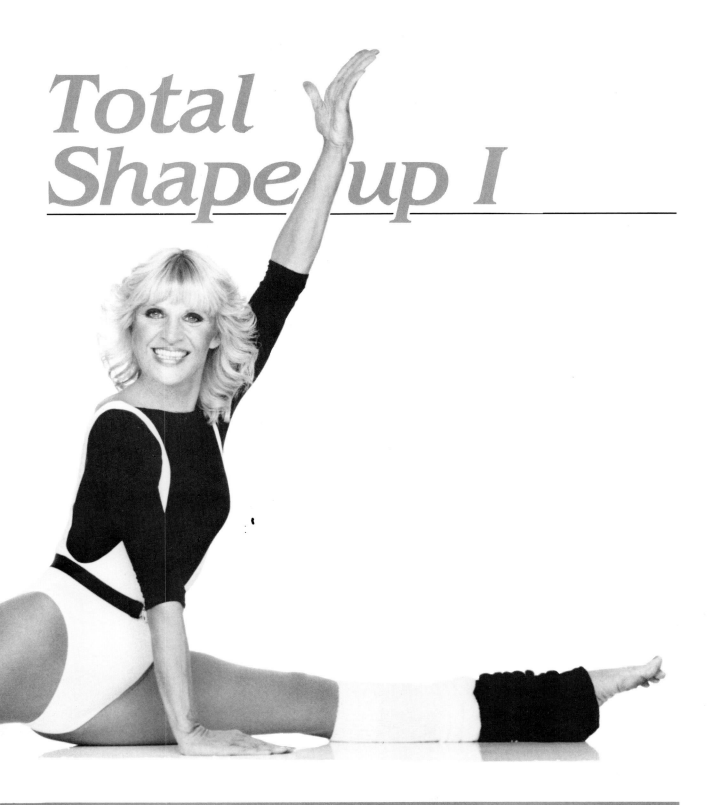

Total Shape-up I
Aerobic Routines for Monday, Wednesday, and Friday

Warm-up—5 Minutes

Leaping into action with cold muscles invites strain, pulling, tearing, even injury to the back. Just as you warm up your car, you should warm up your body before every exercise session.

Effective warm-ups are characterized by *gentle pulsing movements*. Slow static stretches before fast demanding activity aren't good for you. You have to prepare your body for action. You want to lessen stiffness, increase the flow of oxygen and blood, gradually elevate the heart rate, stretch the muscles in different directions.

Choose upbeat music, both to provide a rhythm for your movements and to put you in a moving frame of mind. Remember, a proper warm-up doesn't hold positions; rather it's a series of movements in itself.

LET'S START!

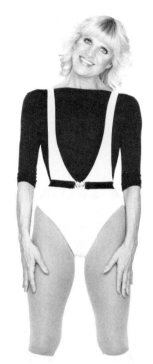

1A

Stand with the legs 2 feet apart, arms relaxed. Gently bring your head to the right. Then . . .

1B

. . . bring it back to the left. Pulse from side to side for a total count of 10 (5 on each side).

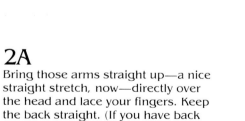

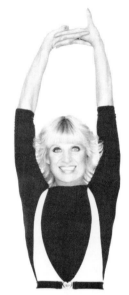

2A

Bring those arms straight up—a nice straight stretch, now—directly over the head and lace your fingers. Keep the back straight. (If you have back problems, soften the knees.) Keep in this position and . . .

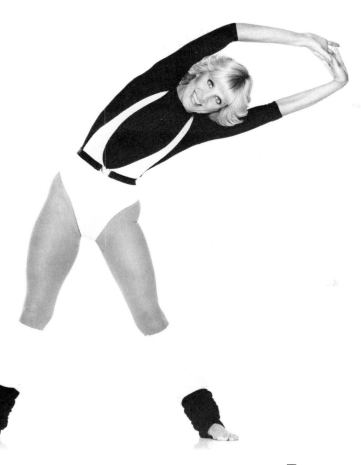

2B

. . . lean to the left. Now pulse *gently* 10 times. Remember: no jerky movements.

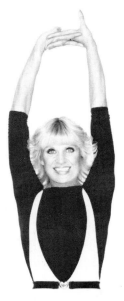

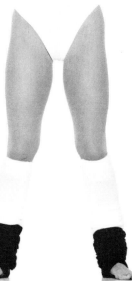

3

Return to position 2A and do 10 gentle pulses to the right.

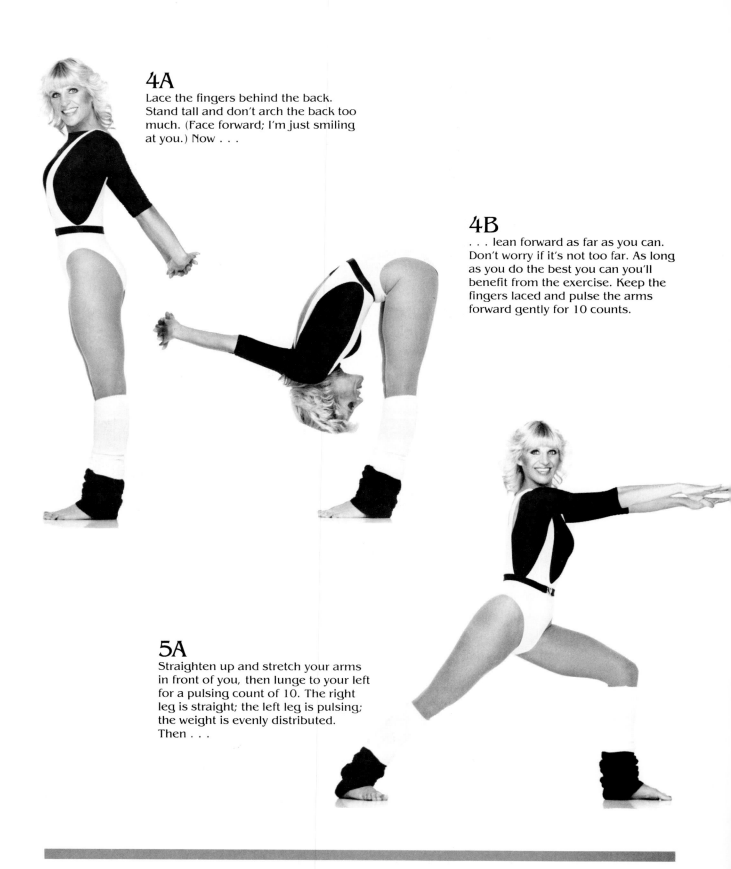

4A

Lace the fingers behind the back. Stand tall and don't arch the back too much. (Face forward; I'm just smiling at you.) Now . . .

4B

. . . lean forward as far as you can. Don't worry if it's not too far. As long as you do the best you can you'll benefit from the exercise. Keep the fingers laced and pulse the arms forward gently for 10 counts.

5A

Straighten up and stretch your arms in front of you, then lunge to your left for a pulsing count of 10. The right leg is straight; the left leg is pulsing; the weight is evenly distributed. Then . . .

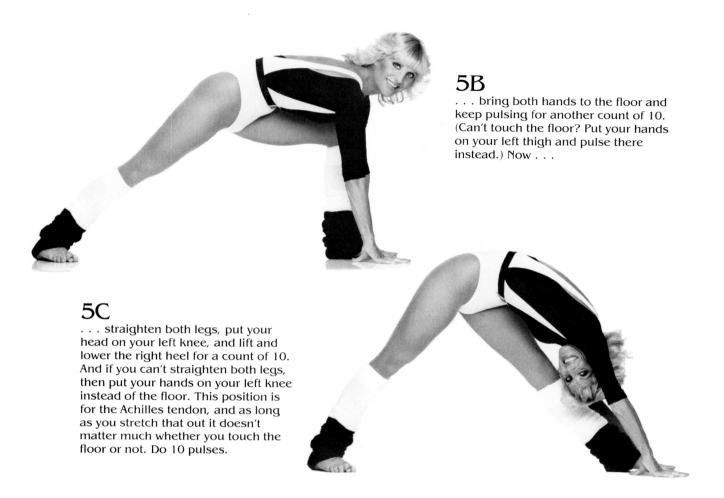

5B

. . . bring both hands to the floor and keep pulsing for another count of 10. (Can't touch the floor? Put your hands on your left thigh and pulse there instead.) Now . . .

5C

. . . straighten both legs, put your head on your left knee, and lift and lower the right heel for a count of 10. And if you can't straighten both legs, then put your hands on your left knee instead of the floor. This position is for the Achilles tendon, and as long as you stretch that out it doesn't matter much whether you touch the floor or not. Do 10 pulses.

REPEAT

Straighten up and repeat 5-A to 5-C, only lunge to your right this time.

Go back to position 1A and repeat the entire routine. Keep going until your 5 minutes are up.

NOTE: Don't forget to chart your progress, by recording your number of repetitions, on this and every routine. If time is up in the middle of a repetition, don't stop. Finish each routine before moving on to the next.

PUT ON YOUR SHOES
It's time for Aerobics—20 Minutes

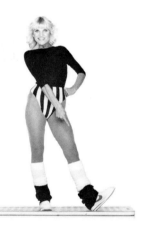

For the next 20 minutes you're going to move and move fast. No bare feet! You need the arch support and cushioning effect of sneakers or running shoes. Remember, the point of aerobics is to get the heart pounding, the blood coursing, and the perspiration flowing. Keep the music fast. (*Not* "The Flight of the Bumble Bee," please, just upbeat!) There's no aerobic benefit unless you work up a sweat.

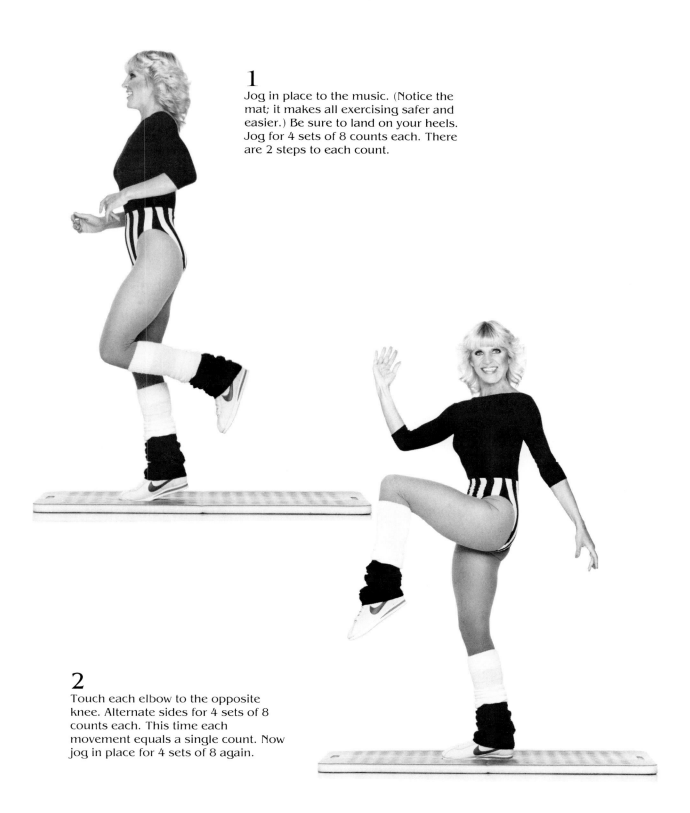

1

Jog in place to the music. (Notice the mat; it makes all exercising safer and easier.) Be sure to land on your heels. Jog for 4 sets of 8 counts each. There are 2 steps to each count.

2

Touch each elbow to the opposite knee. Alternate sides for 4 sets of 8 counts each. This time each movement equals a single count. Now jog in place for 4 sets of 8 again.

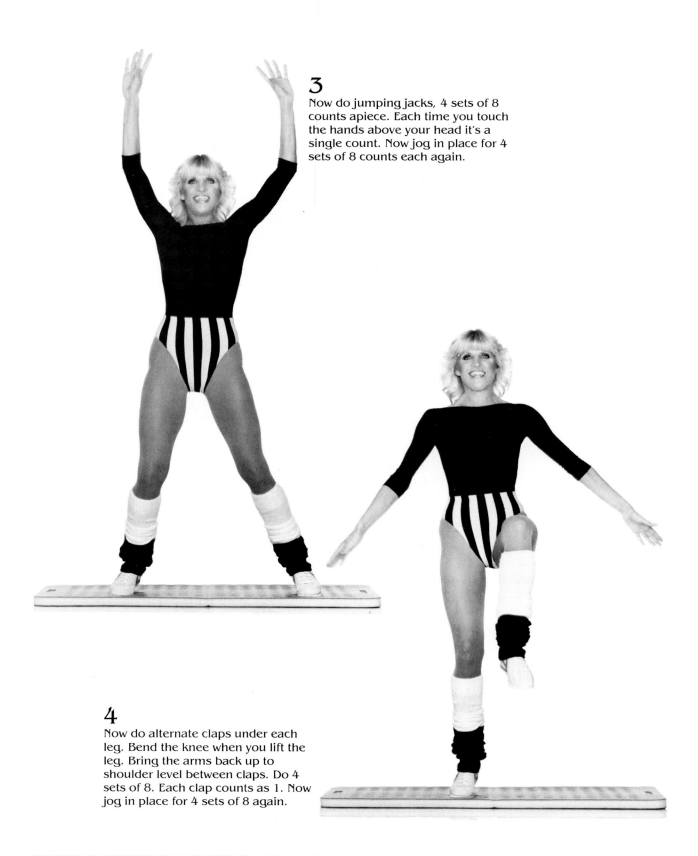

3

Now do jumping jacks, 4 sets of 8 counts apiece. Each time you touch the hands above your head it's a single count. Now jog in place for 4 sets of 8 counts each again.

4

Now do alternate claps under each leg. Bend the knee when you lift the leg. Bring the arms back up to shoulder level between claps. Do 4 sets of 8. Each clap counts as 1. Now jog in place for 4 sets of 8 again.

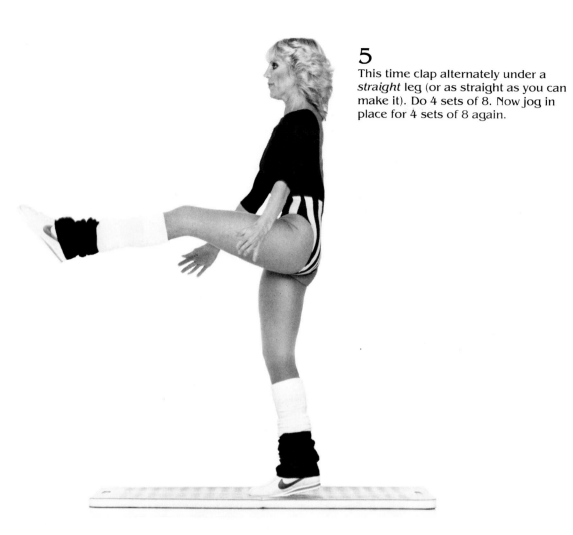

5

This time clap alternately under a *straight* leg (or as straight as you can make it). Do 4 sets of 8. Now jog in place for 4 sets of 8 again.

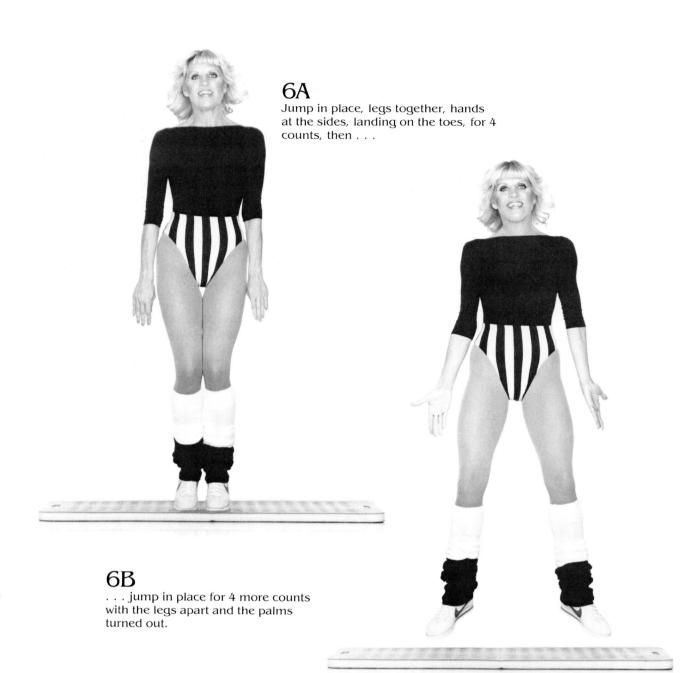

6A
Jump in place, legs together, hands at the sides, landing on the toes, for 4 counts, then . . .

6B
. . . jump in place for 4 more counts with the legs apart and the palms turned out.

REPEAT

Repeat position 6 one more time, then jog in place for 4 sets of 8. Go back to position 1 and repeat the entire routine until your 20 minutes are up.

NOTE: Do what you can. Don't be upset if you can't make it through an exercise or through the whole routine. When anything's too difficult, go back to the jogging. Doing a part of the routine is better than doing none. Your goal is to keep going a full 20 minutes. If you fall short, don't get discouraged. You'll work up to it.

ANOTHER NOTE: Of course, if you just sailed effortlessly through all of this, then start it again. And if 20 minutes runs out in the middle of a repetition, *don't stop in the middle.*

THE LAST NOTE: I won't say it again, but one last time, be *sure* to record the number of repetitions you do of this and every routine on your Progress Chart on page 7.

Instant Side-Stitch Therapy

Everyone who exercises gets side stitches from time to time. They're those sharp sudden pains in the side, usually due either to:

1. an inadequate supply of blood to the diaphragm, which you can relieve simply by slowing down until your body can restore the necessary blood supply; or

2. a small pocket of air trapped in the intestines, which can be alleviated by exhaling forcibly and repeatedly for a minute, bearing down as you exhale as if vigorously clearing the throat.

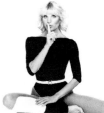

Cool-down—5 Minutes

Especially after an aerobic segment, the body needs time to gear down slowly. You don't want to just slam on the brakes and come to a screeching halt. The purpose of the cool-down is to allow the blood, which during aerobics is concentrated in the legs, to get back to the heart. It's also an opportunity to lengthen out and relax the muscles.

The cool-down is really the icing on the exercise cake. It's a dynamic way to wash out body tension. It'll leave you feeling refreshed and energetic both in body and in mind. This time put on slower, more relaxing music. And instead of the pulsing movements we used in the warm-up, hold each pose for 20 or 30 seconds to really stretch out those muscles.

Use this same cool-down for aerobic and toning days alike.

Warning: You may feel like walking around a little right after aerobics, which is fine (and an excellent time to monitor your working heart rate). But whatever you do, don't dangle your head lower than your heart. With so much blood in the legs you may pass out!

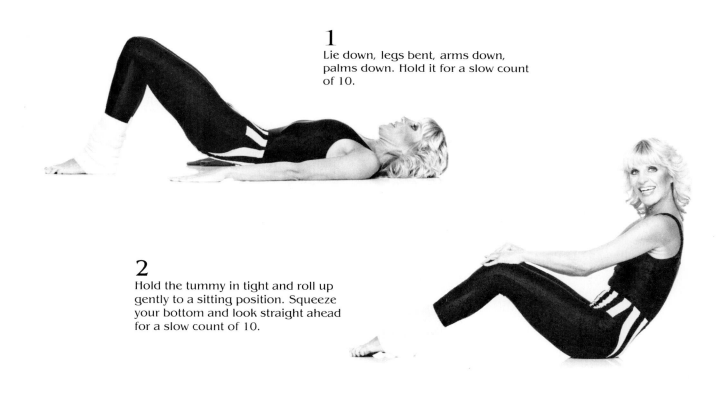

1
Lie down, legs bent, arms down, palms down. Hold it for a slow count of 10.

2
Hold the tummy in tight and roll up gently to a sitting position. Squeeze your bottom and look straight ahead for a slow count of 10.

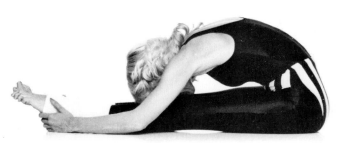

3

Now straighten those legs and bring the head forward to the knee. You want to stretch out those hamstrings for 10 slow counts. (I know this isn't easy. Push forward with the lower spine and do the best you can.)

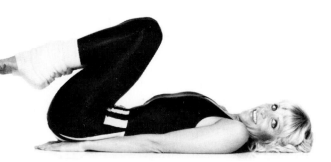

4

Roll your back down flat on the floor, bend the legs, and put your hands palm down underneath your bottom.

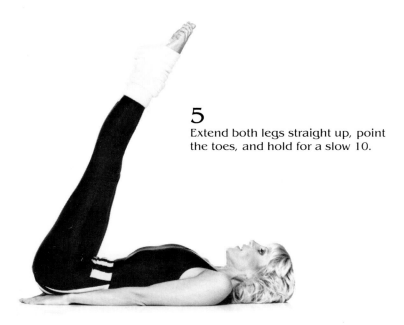

5

Extend both legs straight up, point the toes, and hold for a slow 10.

6

Stay in position 5, but now point the heels instead of the toes. Hold for another slow 10.

7

Lower the legs by bending them first at the knees. Lie flat, toes pointed, tummy held in, and concentrate on pushing your vertebrae flat against the mat. Stay in position for a slow count of 10.

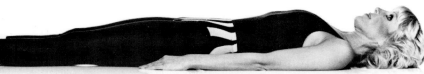

8

Keep in position 7, but this time lift your head up for the slow count to 10.

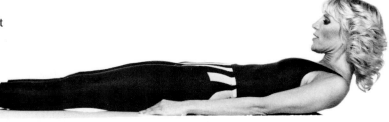

9

Now let the head back down and stretch the arms way back, keeping those vertebrae flat on the ground, please. Tighten the body and pretend somebody is pulling on your fingers and toes for a final slow count of 10. Then release the tension and feel it drain away.

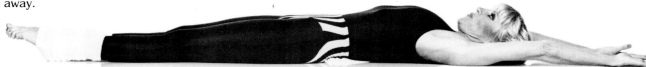

REPEAT

Go back to position 1 and repeat the entire routine. Keep going until your 5 minutes are up.

END OF TODAY'S AEROBIC ROUTINES BYE-BYE!

I'm Exercising but I'm Not Losing Weight!

Muscle weighs more than the same volume of fat. To put it another way, a pound of muscle takes up less room than a pound of fat. So your measurements may shrink even though the scale doesn't budge.

Don't Do It!

Deep knee bends are·one of the *worst* exercises a woman can do. It's not the going down, it's the coming up, when all your body weight is supported by the knees.

Electrode Exercises

There's a new type of machine in certain pricy big-city salons these days. You lie still on a table while someone administers a series of electric shocks to your muscles. Supposedly this will make you look like Burt or Farrah without the slightest effort on your part.

For rehabilitation of the disabled, these machines may have some use. But for able-bodied women and men they are a waste of time—besides being painful and expensive. If you want to build up your body you've got to work out, breathe hard, and sweat. Electric shocks won't do it for you.

Total Shape-up I
Toning Routines for Tuesday and Thursday

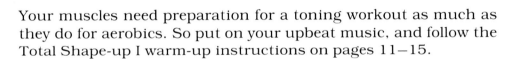

Warm-up—5 Minutes

Your muscles need preparation for a toning workout as much as they do for aerobics. So put on your upbeat music, and follow the Total Shape-up I warm-up instructions on pages 11–15.

The Most Important Thing in Exercise Is . . .
BREATHING

Many people when they concentrate unconsciously hold their breath. Very very bad! Among other things, holding the breath while exercising can cause a dangerous buildup of pressure in the chest and reduce vital blood flow to the brain. Whenever you exercise, *always keep breathing.*

Waist—5 Minutes

In all the waist exercises it's very important to *keep the body straight* and *pulse* it to the sides. Do not jerk back and forth.

To make the exercises more effective, tighten the buttocks and hold the stomach in. Don't slouch and jerk; tighten and pulsate instead. Always think of your posture, lift the ribcage high, and *breathe!* Hold the buttocks, not your breath! Exhale as you move; inhale on the way back.

Besides spare-tire removal, waist exercises have another important benefit—they strengthen the back. People often overlook the fact that abdominal muscles help support the spine. In fact, weak abdominals often contribute to bad backs.

If you've already got a bad back, *always* keep the knees a little bent when doing exercises. Sharp pains mean you're exceeding yourself, so slow down. Even if you can't do the movements completely, whatever you *can* do is *good enough.* Just trying helps.

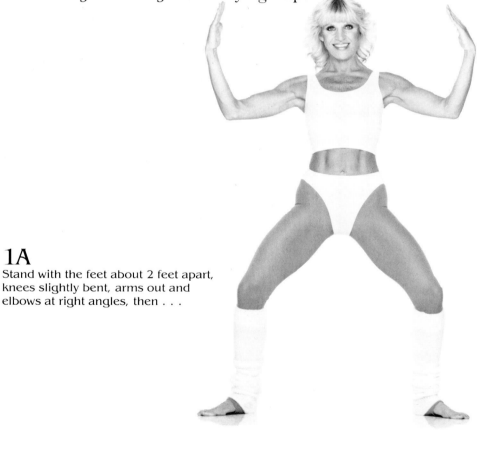

1A
Stand with the feet about 2 feet apart, knees slightly bent, arms out and elbows at right angles, then . . .

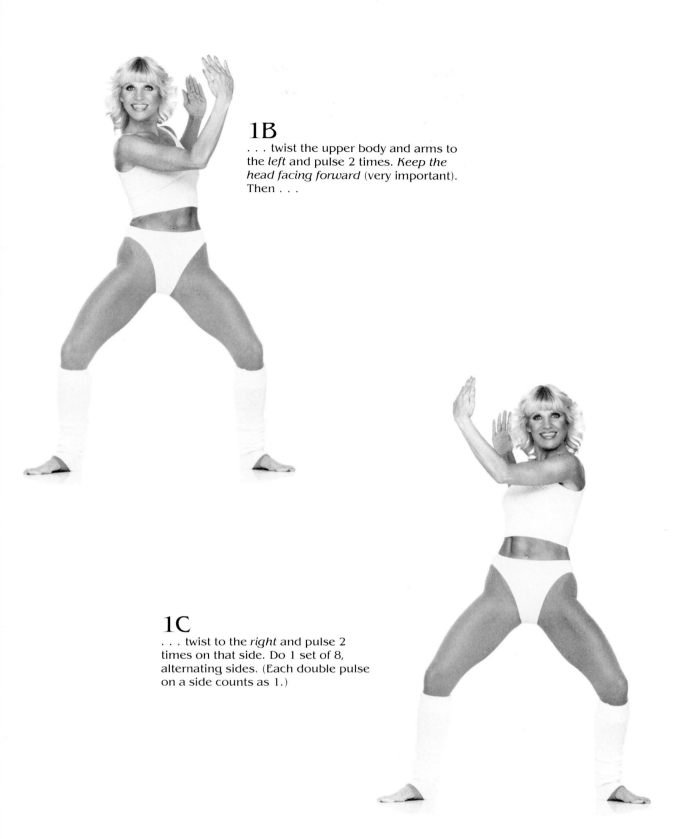

1B

. . . twist the upper body and arms to the *left* and pulse 2 times. *Keep the head facing forward* (very important). Then . . .

1C

. . . twist to the *right* and pulse 2 times on that side. Do 1 set of 8, alternating sides. (Each double pulse on a side counts as 1.)

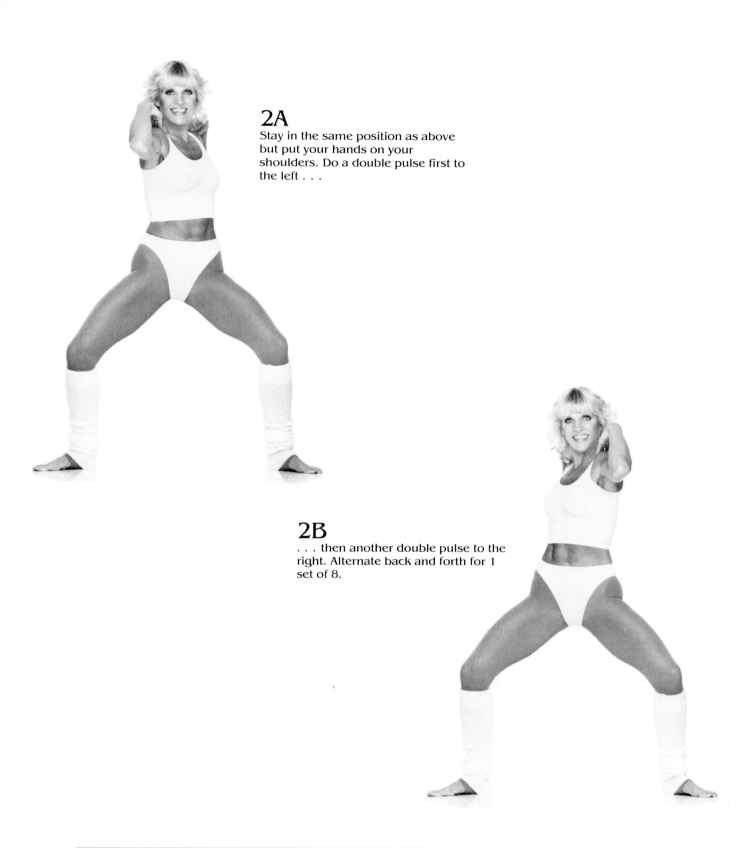

2A
Stay in the same position as above but put your hands on your shoulders. Do a double pulse first to the left . . .

2B
. . . then another double pulse to the right. Alternate back and forth for 1 set of 8.

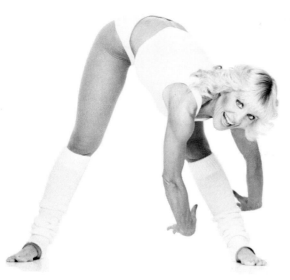

3A

Straighten the legs, keeping the knees soft. Bend over and point the tops of the wrists at the floor and your chin at your knee. Do 2 pulses to the left, wrists on either side of your calf, then . . .

3B

. . . another 2 pulses to the right. Alternate back and forth for 1 set of 8. Don't worry if your body isn't as far forward as mine. Try your best.

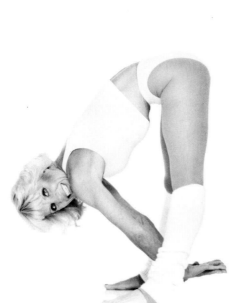

4

This time put both hands between your legs and pulse from the waist for 1 set of 8. (Soften the knees if you have back trouble.)

5A
Stand with legs apart, knees straight, head tucked down, and arms extended. Then . . .

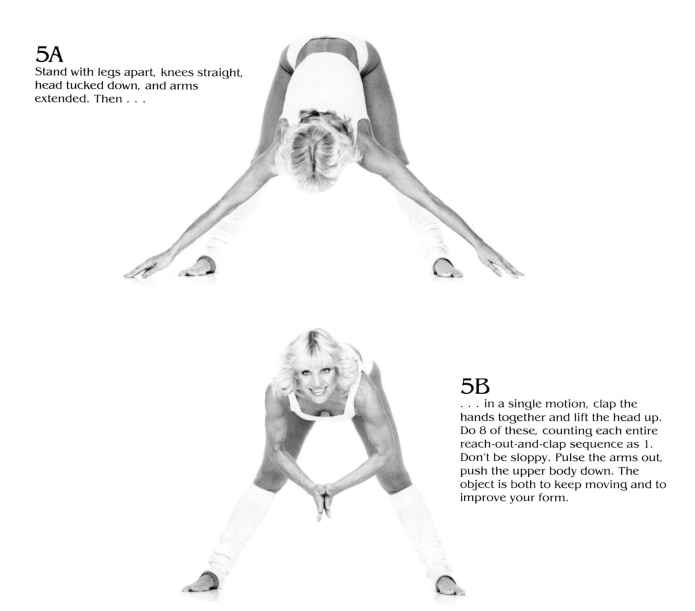

5B
. . . in a single motion, clap the hands together and lift the head up. Do 8 of these, counting each entire reach-out-and-clap sequence as 1. Don't be sloppy. Pulse the arms out, push the upper body down. The object is both to keep moving and to improve your form.

REPEAT

Go back to position 1A and repeat the entire waist routine. Keep going until your 5 minutes are up.

Stomach—5 Minutes

We must attack *three* different stomach muscles. We will tighten *midriff muscles*, site of the unloved "midriff bulge," with moves resembling sit-ups. We'll tone up the *obliques*, known as "love handles," by twisting to the left and right and by touching opposite knees. Finally, we'll condition the *transverse muscles*, the infamous "potbelly," by means of leg lifts.

Flattening the stomach is possible, but it can't be achieved by stomach exercises alone. True, body fat is burned by means of exercise. But it *burns all over the body at an equal rate.* In other words, a good aerobic workout will burn more fat off your midriff than an equal amount of time spent on sit-ups. That's because aerobics get you hotter and therefore burn off more fat. When you exercise the stomach muscles you tone them up, but whatever fat you burn is coming off the *entire body*, not just off the stomach area. That's why we say there's no such thing as spot reducing.

The most effective means to enhance stomach exercises is to keep "thinking the stomach in." Pretend an elephant is stepping on it. This not only strengthens the stomach muscles but makes it easier to sit up too.

Two more things:

1. *Exhale on the way up; inhale on the way down.* Even if it seems backward this helps tone stomach muscles.

2. If your neck gets tired in a pose, reach back and hold the top of your head with your hands.

1A
First, the midriffs. Lie flat, hands behind your head, and . . .

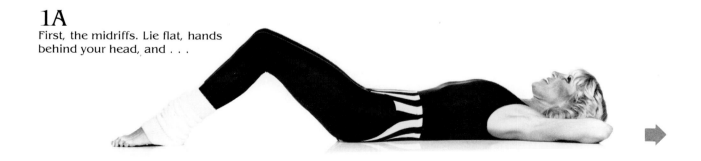

1B

. . . lift the head only. Be sure to keep the elbows back and in line with the ears; the lower back on the ground; the stomach muscles held tight; the face looking upward. Remember to breath *out* on the way up, and *in* on the way down. Seems backward, I know, but this will help the toning effect on the stomach. Do 1 set of 8, counting each time your head touches the floor as 1. (NOTE: If you have trouble putting both hands behind your head, try it with only one hand. If even that is too hard, then keep both hands on your thighs.)

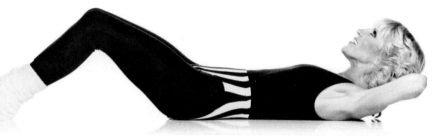

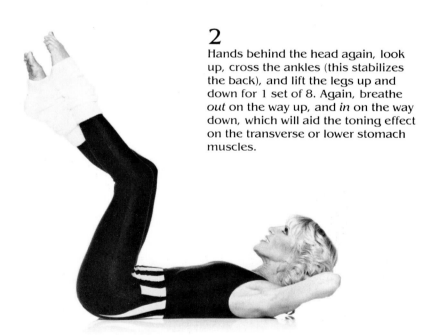

2

Hands behind the head again, look up, cross the ankles (this stabilizes the back), and lift the legs up and down for 1 set of 8. Again, breathe *out* on the way up, and *in* on the way down, which will aid the toning effect on the transverse or lower stomach muscles.

3A

The following sequence is a bicycle movement for the obliques (a.k.a. "love handles"). Lie down, twist to the right, and touch the right elbow to the left knee. Keep the toes pointed and the other leg as straight as possible. Then . . .

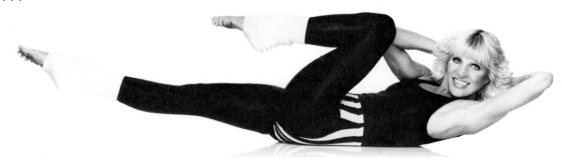

3B

. . . twist in the other direction and touch the left elbow to the right knee. *Remember: Exhale* each time an elbow touches a knee and *inhale* during the twist from side to side. *Keep the lower back on the floor* at all times.

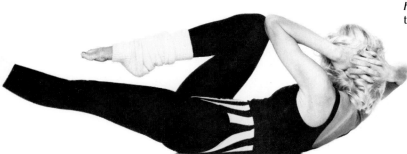

4A

Here's a tough one, but it's a fantastic pot toner and worth the agony. Prop your upper body up on your elbows, keeping the hands under the bottom with the palms down. Face forward, lift the legs, point the toes, and cross the feet, one over the other, for 1 set of 8. Now . . .

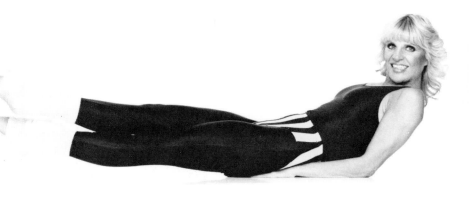

4B

. . . lift the legs higher and do the same crisscross movement for another set of 8.

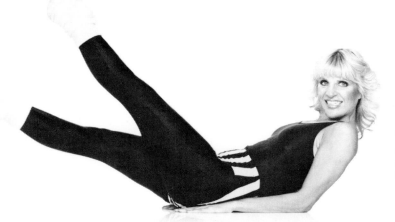

REPEAT

Go back to position 1A and repeat the entire routine. Keep going until your 5 minutes are up.

Arms and Pectorals (Bust)— 5 Minutes

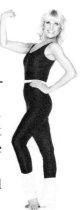

Women's triceps and biceps muscles just seem destined to sag. And to add insult to injury, we have a tendency to accumulate fat there and on our backs as well. Now we're going to work on these muscles and on the pectorals, which lie beneath the bust.

About that bust, appealing as we all know it is, let's not kid ourselves about what it's made of. Busts are just fat and glands. They get bigger when you gain weight, get pregnant, or have an implant. Exotic squeezing devices and special bust-enlarging exercises don't work. You can't expect muscle-building techniques to do anything unless you've got a muscle to build!

Firming up underlying pectorals may add a little to the bustline. But not much. Toning up biceps and triceps will counteract the drapery effect under the arms. But not if you've recently lost 40 or 50 pounds. In that case those hanging triceps muscles may be just loose skin.

The following exercises will actually tone and strengthen the entire upper body. They'll be more effective with 3-to-5-pound weights held in each hand. But whether you use weights or not, whenever you lift your arms, *always keep them up at shoulder level.* And don't hunch the shoulders; keep them relaxed.

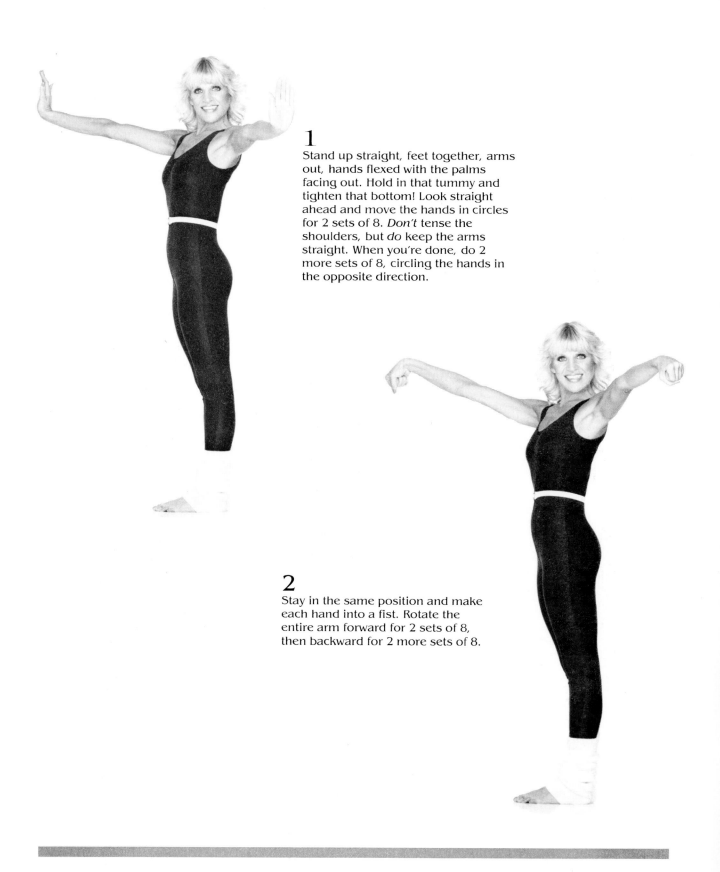

1

Stand up straight, feet together, arms out, hands flexed with the palms facing out. Hold in that tummy and tighten that bottom! Look straight ahead and move the hands in circles for 2 sets of 8. *Don't* tense the shoulders, but *do* keep the arms straight. When you're done, do 2 more sets of 8, circling the hands in the opposite direction.

2

Stay in the same position and make each hand into a fist. Rotate the entire arm forward for 2 sets of 8, then backward for 2 more sets of 8.

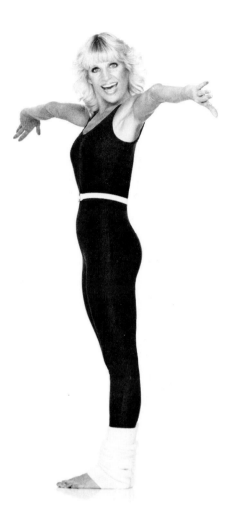

3
Again remain in position, but this time extend the fingers and twist the palms up to face the ceiling. Circle first one way, then the other. Do 2 sets of 8, counting each double movement as 1.

4A
Bring the arms forward, elbows at shoulder level, until one hand covers the other. (NOTE: Bending the knee is *optional*. Do it to relax your back only if you want or need to.) Then . . .

4B
. . . pulse the elbows back. Do 2 sets of 8.

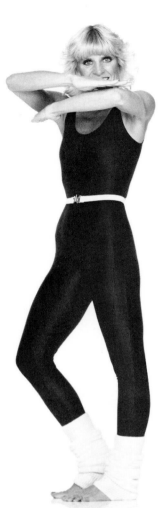

5A
This time bring the arms in closer, hand above the elbow, knee bent if it's more comfortable, face forward, and . . .

5B
. . . fling both arms fully out. Keep the movement controlled and the arms at shoulder level. Do 2 sets of 8.

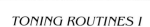

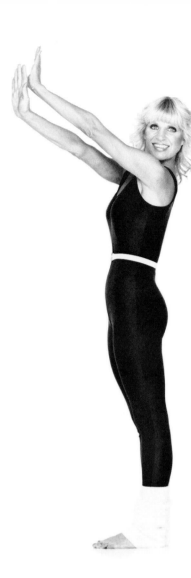

6A

Bring the feet together (if they've been apart), face forward again, (*not like me!*) flex the hands, and push the palms up and out in front of you. Cross the flexed hands, then . . .

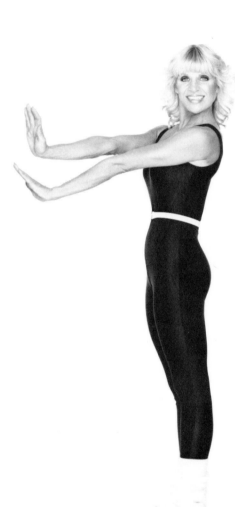

6B

. . . lower the arms and cross them the other way. Each complete crisscross-up-and-crisscross-down counts 1. Do 2 sets of 8.

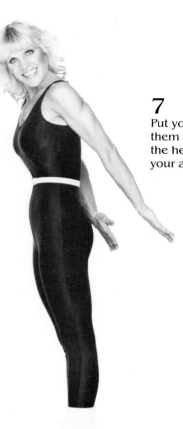

7

Put your arms behind your back, hold them out from your bottom, and keep the head forward and straight. Cross your arms behind you for 2 sets of 8.

REPEAT

Go back to position 1 and repeat the entire routine. Keep going until your 5 minutes are up.

The Euphoria Hormone

Vigorous workouts boast an unusual side effect —namely, a subtle but deeply pleasurable feeling of well-being that lasts for hours after your exercise session. The feeling is literally habit-forming. It stems from the release into the bloodstream of narcotic-like substances called endorphins during periods of physical activity. The more you exercise, the more addicted to the effect you become. In fact, the unconscious craving for endorphins helps *keep* you exercising regularly.

Thighs—5 Minutes

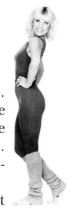

This and the routine for hips that follows are just plain tough. Sorry, there's nothing I can do about it. Go through this exercise as fast as you can, and be sure to do all the repetitions on one side *before* switching to the other. Don't alternate back and forth. You need to work up a lot of tiring heat to burn off that intermuscular fat.

It doesn't feel great, I know. Especially the part of your leg that faces the ceiling. But keep at it.

1

Lie on your right side, propped on the right elbow. Lean forward a bit on the pelvis. The right leg is bent back for balance and the *left toe is pointed.* Now lift the left leg in a pulsing motion up and down for 2 sets of 8. Don't worry if you can't get it as high as mine; at least 12 inches off the ground is enough.

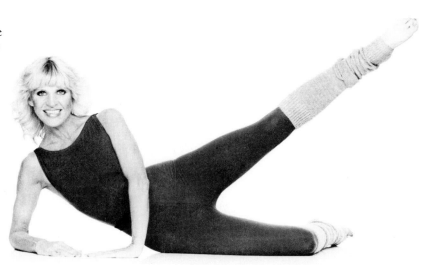

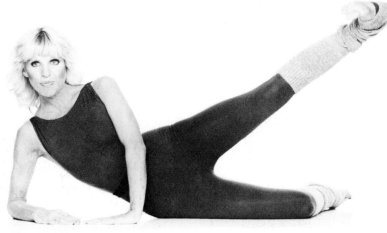

2
This time *flex the left foot forward* and do the same up-and-down pulsing movement with the leg for another 2 sets of 8.

3
Now bring the left leg in front of you, foot still pointed. The left arm goes up and back for balance. Lift the left leg up and down 12 inches for 2 sets of 8. (NOTE: *Don't* let the left leg touch the floor!)

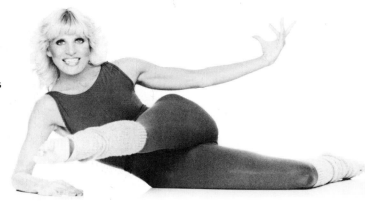

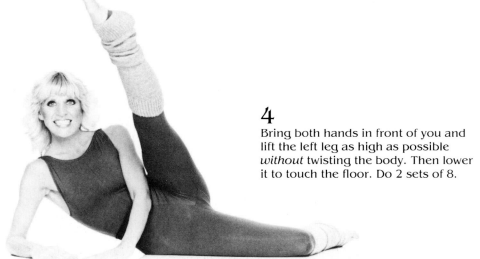

4
Bring both hands in front of you and lift the left leg as high as possible *without* twisting the body. Then lower it to touch the floor. Do 2 sets of 8.

5A
Bend both legs back at the knee and . . .

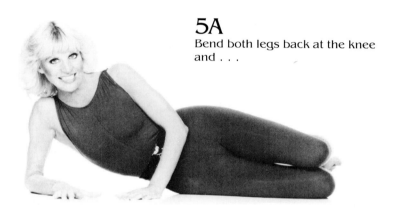

5B
. . . lift and lower the top leg for 2 sets of 8. Don't think of the pain. Focus instead on those cottage-cheese bulges you'll soon banish from the sides of your thighs. (NOTE: It's very important to keep the *side* of the thigh facing the ceiling. Be sure the foot goes up at the same time the knee does.)

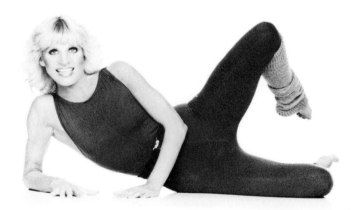

6

Bring the left leg over the right leg. Then either grasp the left ankle or if it's more comfortable put both hands on the floor. Flex the right foot (heel down, toe up) and lift the *right* (lower) leg up and down off the floor for 2 sets of 8. (NOTE: And be sure again that the inner thigh faces the ceiling.)

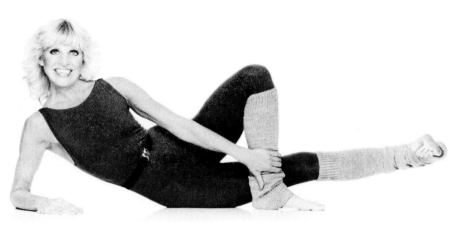

REPEAT

Go back to position 1 and repeat the entire routine on the other side. Keep going until your 5 minutes are up.

Leg Warmers Soothe Tired Leg Muscles

When you do exercises, your muscles produce a waste product called lactic acid. This substance is what causes muscular soreness and stiffness. The body's normal blood flow eventually washes away lactic acids. If you keep the leg muscles warm with leg warmers, then the blood flow to that area will be increased and the level of lactic acid will be more efficiently reduced. As a result you'll feel less stiffness and soreness in the legs.

Hips—5 Minutes

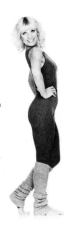

Hips are more of the same misery as thighs. If it's any comfort to you, most people find leg routines toughest.

Quick relief: If you get too tired doing this or the thigh series, try the following simple maneuver. Get down on all fours; breathe calmly; let the head dangle; keep the arms straight at the elbows. Now sit back on your heels for a moment; come back slowly to all fours and just stay that way, elbows still straight, until you feel ready to continue.

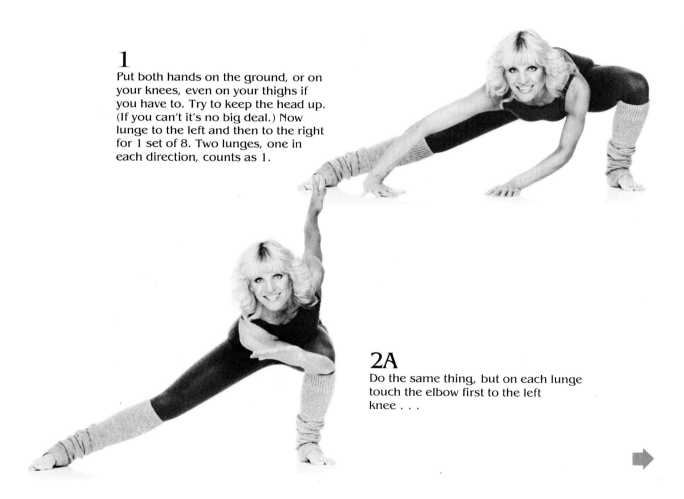

1
Put both hands on the ground, or on your knees, even on your thighs if you have to. Try to keep the head up. (If you can't it's no big deal.) Now lunge to the left and then to the right for 1 set of 8. Two lunges, one in each direction, counts as 1.

2A
Do the same thing, but on each lunge touch the elbow first to the left knee . . .

2B

. . . and then to the right knee. Or to whatever you *can* touch. Do 1 set of 8.

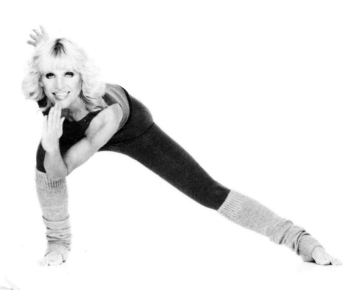

3A

This time try to get the elbow first all the way down to your left ankle . . .

3B

. . . and then all the way down to the right ankle. Or as far down as you can. Do 1 set of 8.

4A

For your final lunges, extend the right arm first out past the left foot . . .

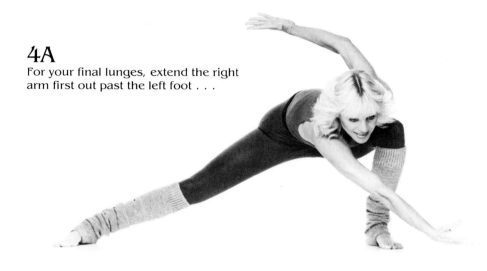

4B

. . . and then the left arm out past the right foot. Again do 1 set of 8.

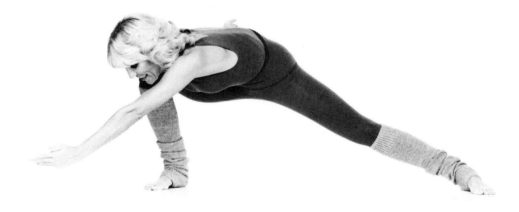

5

Now do the frog. Feet are *parallel;* head faces *forward* (*not* like me!). Don't bounce or jerk, but pulse up and down like a frog on a lily pad for 1 set of 8.

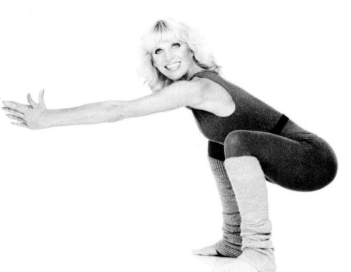

REPEAT

Go back to position 1 and repeat the entire routine. Keep going until your 5 minutes are up.

Women Lose Weight from the Head Down

There's a good chance that even after you reach your ideal weight the sight of your hips may still drive you to tears. That's because female hips and thighs seem to be the last areas to shed excessive fat. Many women must resign themselves to working an additional *six months* before their new weight is evenly distributed and balanced. Often they must tolerate a drawn face while achieving a total look.

Bottom—5 Minutes

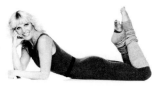

It's not called the gluteus maximus for nothing. It happens to be the biggest muscle in the entire body. And after the age of 20, it starts heading for the feet. You *have* to exercise it . . . or else. These routines are all designed to lift it up—like push-ups for the bottom. Need I add that well-toned gluteals are good for the back? They aid in support of the spine.

Modest suggestion: The simplest and one of the most effective exercises for the gluteals is as elementary as squeezing and holding it—or them. Pretend there's a $100 bill back there. *Then* how long would you hold it?

1
Get on your hands and knees, face forward. (Why am I always looking at the camera? Because I always wanted the models in exercise books to look at me and smile!) Lift the left leg up, *foot flexed,* hold it for a second, then pulse it upward another 6 inches. Push that heel up. Do 2 sets of 8.

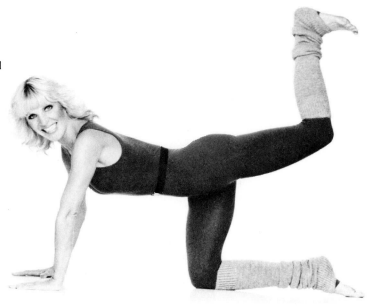

2

Do another 2 sets of 8, this time with
the *toe* pointed up.

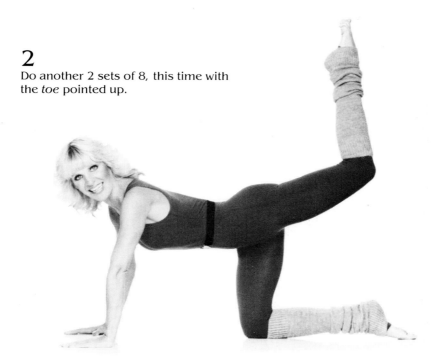

3A

Bring the head down onto or beside
your folded arms. Then . . .

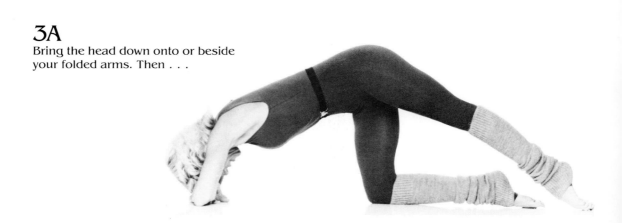

3B

. . . kick the left leg up, toe pointed, for 2 sets of 8.

4

Stay in the same position and kick your bottom with a flexed heel for 2 sets of 8.

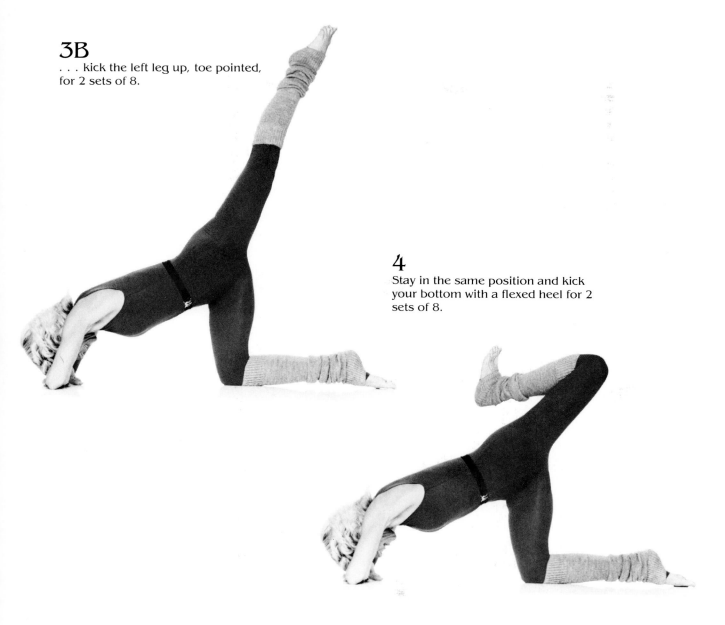

REPEAT

Go back to position 1 and repeat the entire routine with the other leg. Keep going until your 5 minutes are up. Be sure to do the same number of repetitions on both legs before moving on.

Cool-down—5 Minutes

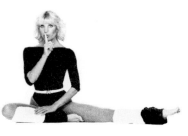

Do the Total Shape-up I cool-down routine described on pages 21–25. *Don't skip it!* Savor the virtuousness of having done all these exercises! Put on soothing music and remember to hold the poses and stretch out those muscles.

END OF TODAY'S TONING ROUTINES BYE-BYE!

Total Shape-up II

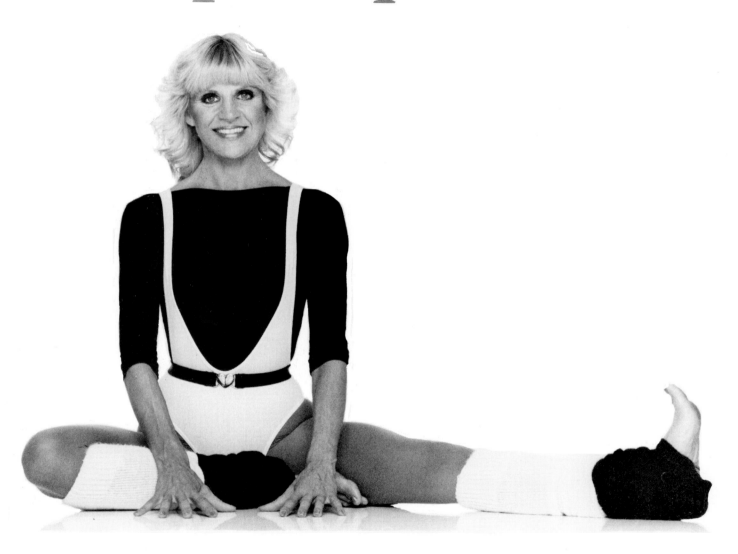

Total Shape-up II
Aerobic Routines for Monday, Wednesday, and Friday

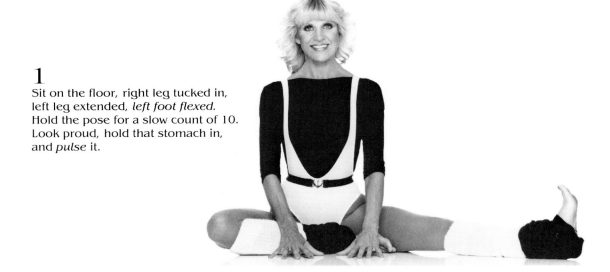

Warm-up—5 Minutes

Three exercise-packed months have now passed, I presume—unless you're using a different calendar than I do. In your Total Shape-up II, the routines will be just a little different, even the warm-up. So put on that upbeat music and remember to *pulse!*

1
Sit on the floor, right leg tucked in, left leg extended, *left foot flexed.* Hold the pose for a slow count of 10. Look proud, hold that stomach in, and *pulse* it.

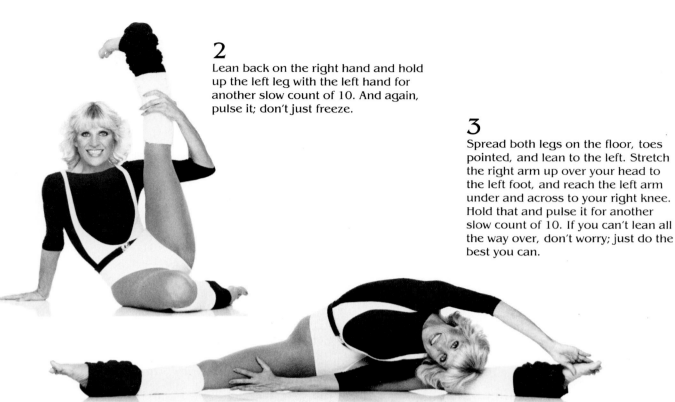

2
Lean back on the right hand and hold up the left leg with the left hand for another slow count of 10. And again, pulse it; don't just freeze.

3
Spread both legs on the floor, toes pointed, and lean to the left. Stretch the right arm up over your head to the left foot, and reach the left arm under and across to your right knee. Hold that and pulse it for another slow count of 10. If you can't lean all the way over, don't worry; just do the best you can.

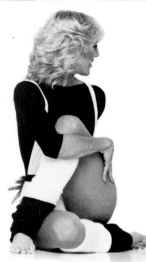

4
Now sit up for a spinal twist. Put the left foot over the right knee, the right arm around the left knee, and turn your head to the left. Hold for 10 slow pulsing counts.

REPEAT

Go back to position 1 and repeat the entire routine on the other side. Keep going until your 5 minutes are up. This is the warm-up you'll use for both aerobic and toning days during Total Shape-up II.

PUT ON YOUR SHOES
It's time for Aerobics—20 Minutes

Keep that music up-tempo. Here come 20 minutes of new aerobic routines. And if you can go a little longer, then by all means do. And don't forget to *wear running shoes!*

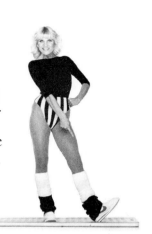

1

Let's have a nice peppy jog for 4 sets of 8. (Right and left together count as 1.) Make sure your heel hits the mat with each step; don't run on your toes.

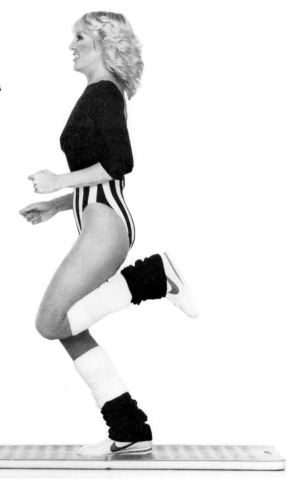

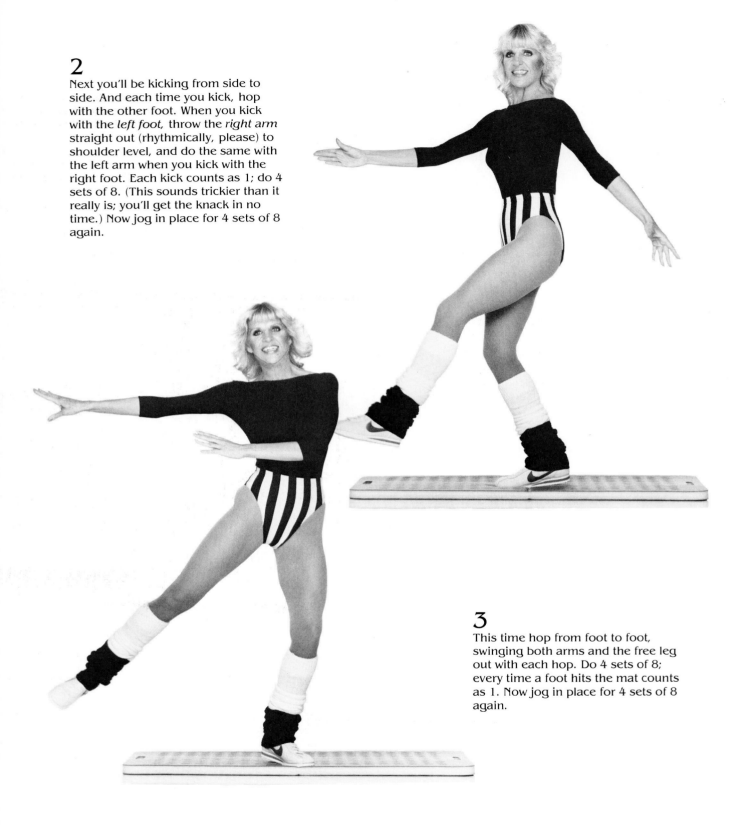

2

Next you'll be kicking from side to side. And each time you kick, hop with the other foot. When you kick with the *left foot,* throw the *right arm* straight out (rhythmically, please) to shoulder level, and do the same with the left arm when you kick with the right foot. Each kick counts as 1; do 4 sets of 8. (This sounds trickier than it really is; you'll get the knack in no time.) Now jog in place for 4 sets of 8 again.

3

This time hop from foot to foot, swinging both arms and the free leg out with each hop. Do 4 sets of 8; every time a foot hits the mat counts as 1. Now jog in place for 4 sets of 8 again.

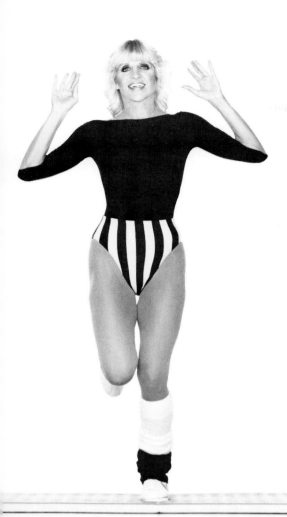

4A

Now you're going to jog with elbows
down on the *left* foot . . .

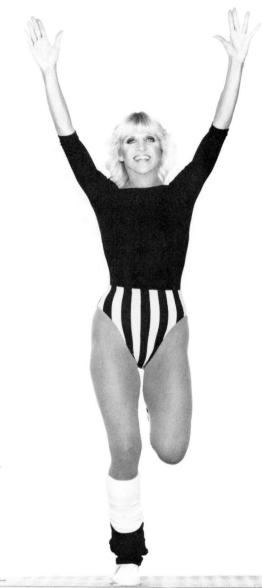

4B

. . . and elbows *up* on the *right* foot.
Do 4 sets of 8. Again, each time a
foot hits the mat it counts as 1.

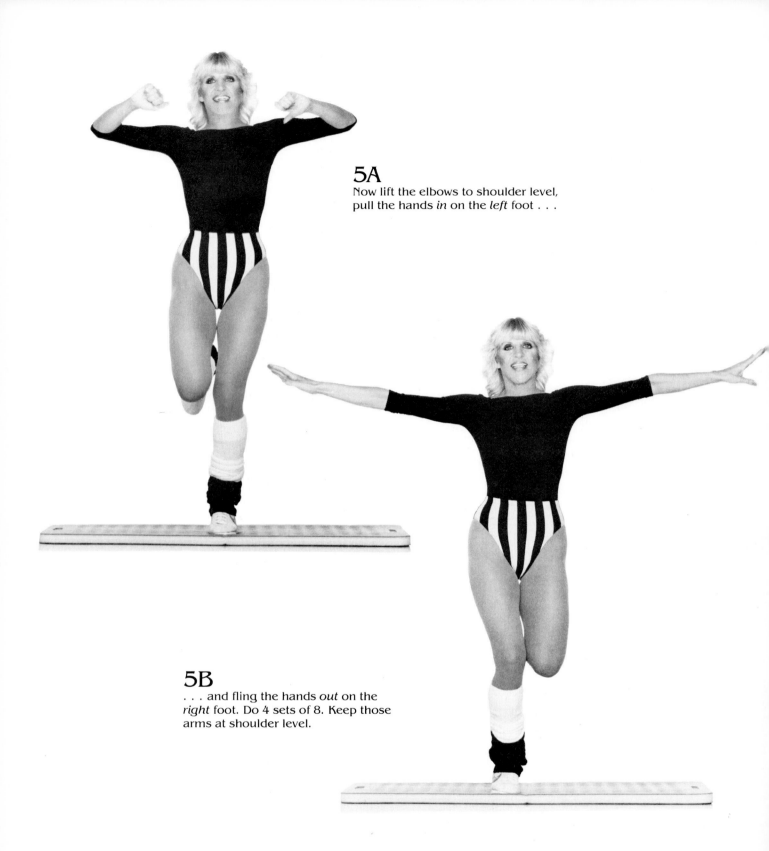

5A
Now lift the elbows to shoulder level, pull the hands *in* on the *left* foot . . .

5B
. . . and fling the hands *out* on the *right* foot. Do 4 sets of 8. Keep those arms at shoulder level.

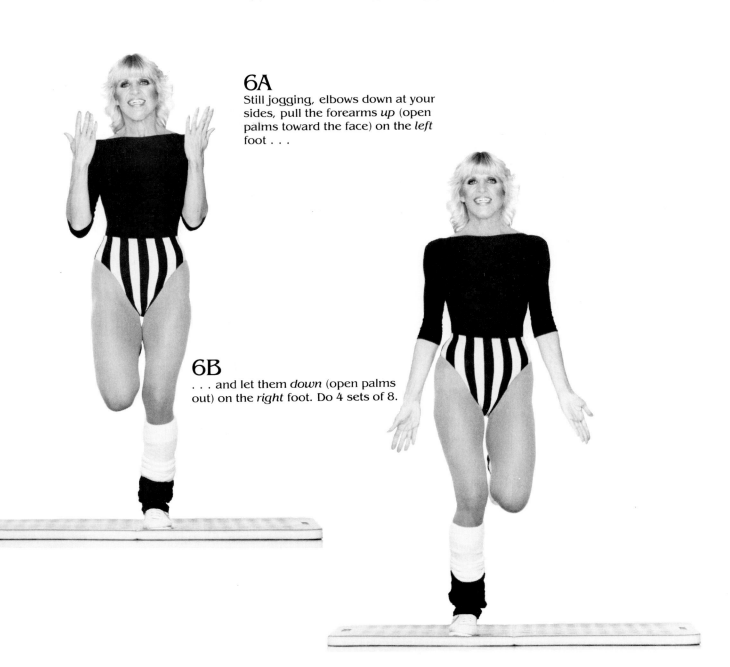

6A
Still jogging, elbows down at your sides, pull the forearms *up* (open palms toward the face) on the *left* foot . . .

6B
. . . and let them *down* (open palms out) on the *right* foot. Do 4 sets of 8.

REPEAT

Go back to position 1 and repeat the entire routine. Keep going until your 20 minutes are up.

Cool-down—5 Minutes

Use this same cool-down for aerobic and toning days alike. Some soothing music, please.

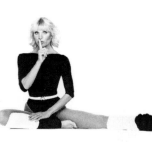

1
Lie down and hug the left knee for a slow count of 10. Toe pointing is optional. And unless you have someone to smile at, look straight ahead at your knee.

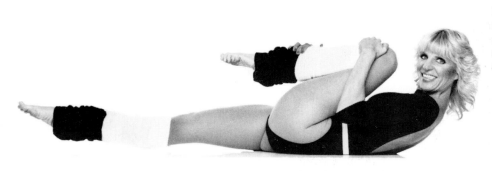

2
Hug the right knee for another slow count of 10.

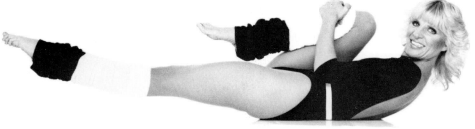

3
Now hug both knees for a slow count of 10.

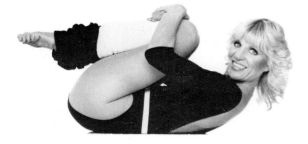

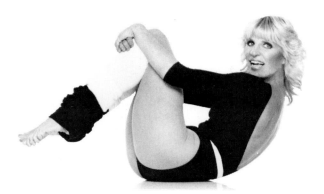

4

Starting in position 3, roll *slowly* forward on the spine until your feet *almost* touch the mat. Then roll slowly back until your *head* almost touches the mat. Go back and forth slowly a total of 10 times.

5

Now stretch the legs straight out, feet flexed as if you were reaching back with your toes. Stretch the hands out and forward, keeping the arms parallel with the legs. Don't hunch, and keep the head up and look forward. Hold (remember: no pulsing in the cool-down) for a slow count of 10.

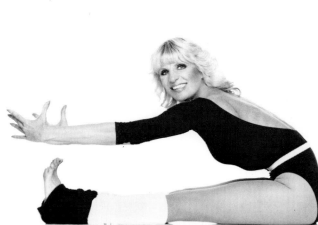

6

Now for the hamstring stretch. Bring the head as close to the knees as possible. Don't be discouraged if you don't fold neatly in half. *Any* attempt will have a positive effect. Flex the toes back and hold for a slow count of 10.

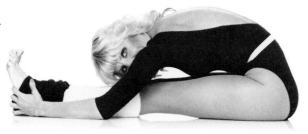

7A

Lie back, bend the legs at the knees, and move them to the *right.* At the same time, put your arms above your head and move them and it to the *left.* Hold for a slow count of 10, then . . .

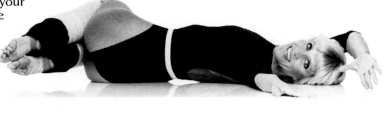

7B

. . . do it the other way, knees to the left, arms and head to the right, for another slow count of 10. Be sure to *keep the shoulders on the floor.* This, by the way, is a fabulous spine release.

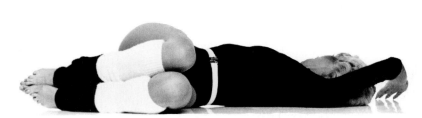

REPEAT

Go back to position 1 and repeat the entire routine. Keep going until your 5 minutes are up.

END OF TODAY'S AEROBIC ROUTINES BYE-BYE!

How to Combat Heat Rash

Inflamed and bumpy skin during a hot day's workout might be a matter of blocked sweat ducts, also known as heat rash. Try cooling off with a shower, powdering the affected area to keep it dry, and applying a bit of calamine lotion.

Sunburn Surprise

Many foods and medicines can make you so sensitive to sunlight that they provoke painful and surprising burns.

Commonly ingested culprits include diet sodas, birth-control pills, tetracycline (the anti-acne medicine), diuretics, and many anti-tension medications.

The biggest problem makers when spilled or applied to sun-exposed skin include the juice of lemons or limes and oil of bergamot (an ingredient in most perfumes).

Beware all of the above whenever you go in the sun.

The Food That Makes Hair Thicker

Hair loss may be inevitable for certain people, but there *is* something you can do for the hair you've got. Namely, you can *thicken* the individual hair shafts with . . . plain unflavored gelatin!

A recent study showed that hair-shaft diameter increased by 45% over a two-month period during which subjects ate a daily dietary supplement of 7 teaspoons of unflavored gelatin. Is thick hair healthy hair? You bet. It's far more manageable and looks better too. When the gelatin was discontinued, everybody's hair reverted to original girth in six months.

Total Shape-up II
Toning Routines for Tuesday and Thursday

Warm-up—5 Minutes

Instructions for your Total Shape-up II warm-up appear on pages 57–58. Really *pulse* to your music!

Waist—5 Minutes

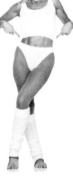

1

Stand with legs 2 feet apart, toes out, knees bent, arms and hands as shown. Pulse to the *left* for 1 set of 8. Keep the hips *still,* and the upper arm *close to the ear.*

2
Keep in position 1 but reach both arms up and point the fingers. Keep leaning left and do 8 more pulses. *Don't* jerk; *don't* straighten the knees.

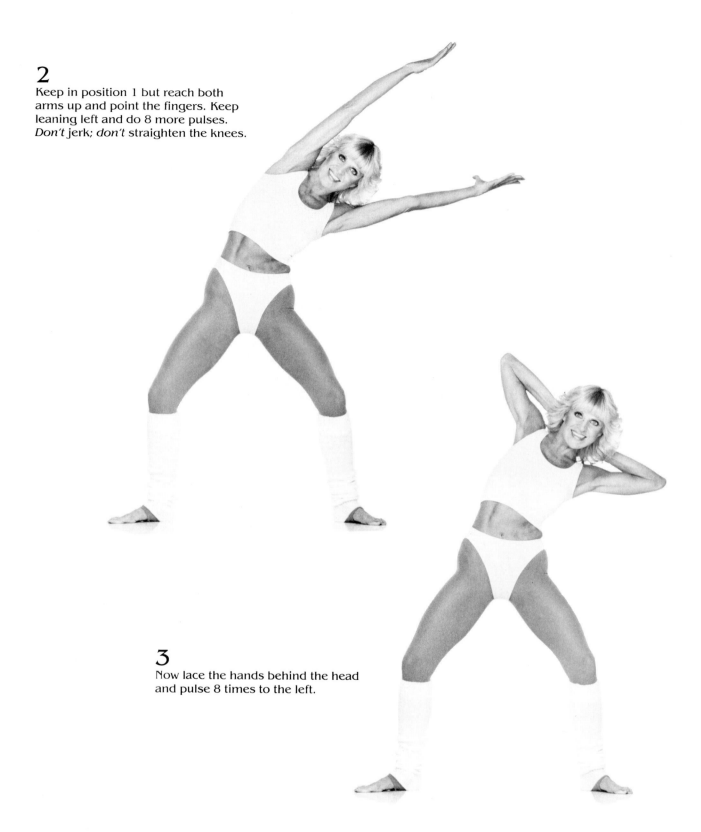

3
Now lace the hands behind the head and pulse 8 times to the left.

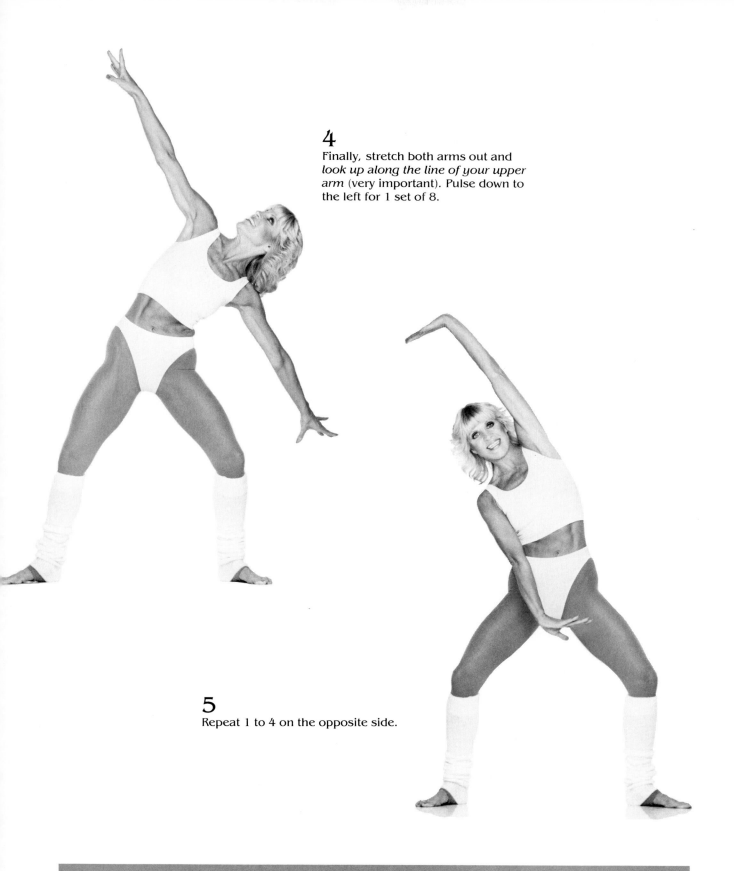

4

Finally, stretch both arms out and *look up along the line of your upper arm* (very important). Pulse down to the left for 1 set of 8.

5

Repeat 1 to 4 on the opposite side.

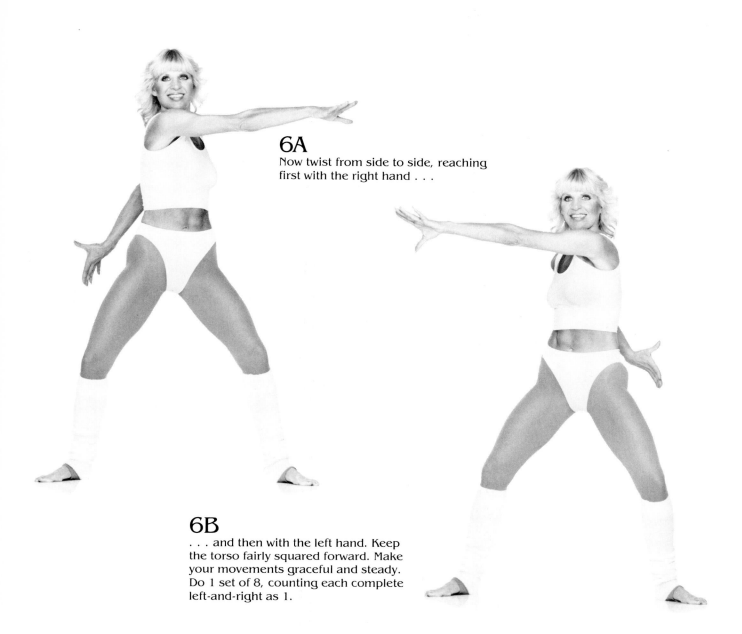

6A
Now twist from side to side, reaching
first with the right hand . . .

6B
. . . and then with the left hand. Keep
the torso fairly squared forward. Make
your movements graceful and steady.
Do 1 set of 8, counting each complete
left-and-right as 1.

REPEAT

Go back to position 1 and repeat the entire waist routine.
Keep going until your 5 minutes are up.

Stronger Bones

Osteoporosis is the clinical name for the softening of the bones that can lead to painful breaks and fractures and a progressive stooping that results from spinal bones so riddled with holes that they collapse into a curve. The condition is the result of calcium deficiency.

To help avoid it, cut down on junk and processed food, much of which contains high levels of phosphorus, a mineral that can block calcium from reaching the bones.

More Tips for Stronger Bones

Cut down on protein. Too much protein in the diet hampers the ability of your kidneys to reabsorb calcium in the bloodstream.

Take a calcium supplement. Many nutritional experts agree that the U.S. government's Recommended Daily Allowance of calcium is 30% too low for women, and that 800 milligrams of calcium per day is closer to what you need.

Exercise. Studies show that women who exercise regularly have thicker, stronger bones.

Help for People Who Can't Digest Milk

OK, so you think this is a pretty small group. That doesn't help if you happen to belong to it. And as a matter of fact, more people than you may think are physically unable to digest milk. They get cramps, bloat, and diarrhea. Worse luck too, since milk is a primary source of calcium, the anti-osteoporosis mineral in which most women are deficient, whether they realize it or not.

Fortunately there is a *new product* on the market called lactaid lactase. Available in pharmacies and some supermarkets (where it's pre-mixed with the milk), it is an enzyme that splits lactose into two easily digestible sugars, glucose and galactose. Result: easily digestible milk.

Stomach—5 Minutes

1

Let's get those obliques: Hands on opposite shoulders, knees bent, back flat on the floor, face forward. Come halfway up (to position shown), *exhaling* as you rise. Then *inhale* as you lower your head back to the floor. Go up and down for 1 set of 8.

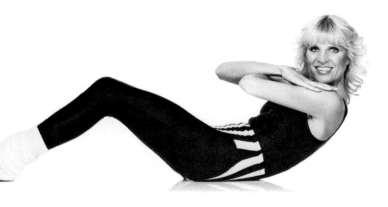

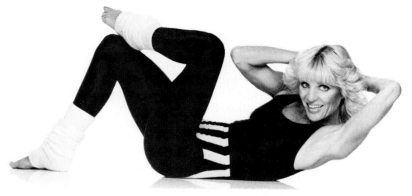

2

Also for the obliques: Lace the hands behind the head, rest the left foot on the right knee, come halfway up (remember to *exhale*), and try to touch the *right elbow* to the *left knee*. On the way down, *inhale* and try *not* to touch the head to the floor. Do 1 set of 8.

3

One more time for the obliques: Stay essentially in position 2 but extend the left leg. Try to touch the right elbow to the left knee, coming up on the exhale and going down *almost* to the floor on the inhale. Do 1 set of 8.

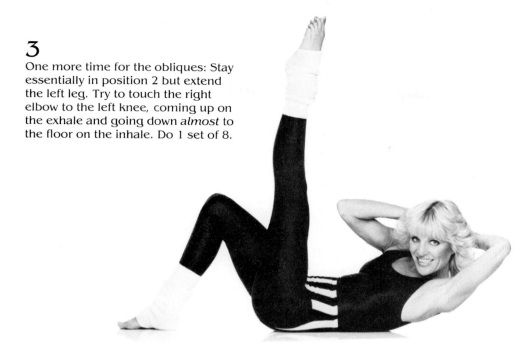

4

Repeat 2 and 3 with the other leg.

5

Now for the midriff: Lie flat on your back, left leg up and bent at the knee, toes pointed. Sit up toward the raised knee, arms on either side of it as shown, face forward (as *not* shown!), and then lie back. Do 8 sit-ups.

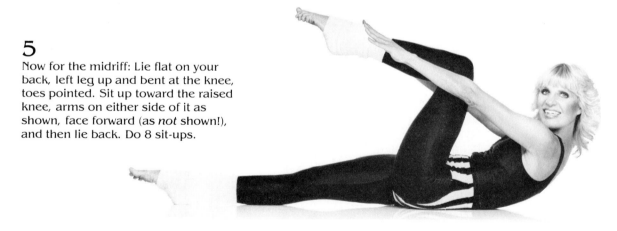

6

Repeat 5 with the right leg up.

7A

This time spread the legs wide apart, lie back with the arms stretched straight above the head, then . . .

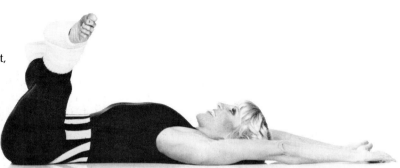

7B

. . . roll smoothly forward and extend the arms between the legs. Then roll back. Do 1 set of 8. Remember to exhale up and inhale down. (Enough of this and soon it'll be goodbye potbelly forever.)

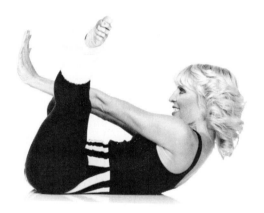

8A

This time, when you sit forward put the arms around the *left* leg for 1 set of 8. And when you're done . . .

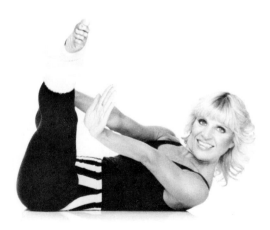

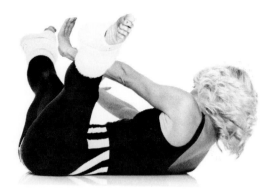

8B
. . . do another set of 8 with your arms around the right leg.

REPEAT

Go back to position 1 and repeat the entire routine. Keep going until your 5 minutes are up.

The More You Exercise, the Easier It Is to Lose Weight

If you exercise four or five times each week, you can lose weight *three times faster* than if you exercise two or three times a week.

Crash Diets

Many people think that slimming down by means of a crash diet will give them more energy. Not true. You can't expect to feel energetic by eliminating essential nutrients.

Arms and Pectorals (Bust)— 5 Minutes

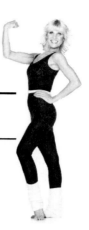

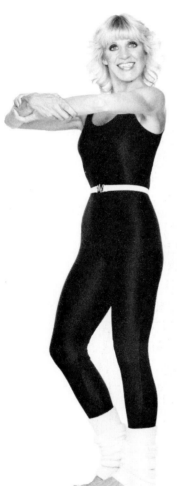

1A

Stand with the feet together (it's *optional* to bend one leg, if you need a little rest), grasp the elbows in front of you, and . . .

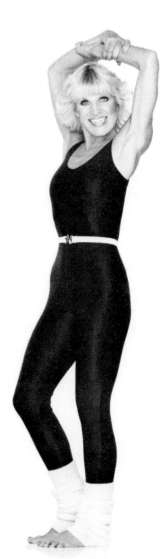

1B

. . . lift them up and down. Do 2 sets of 8; each complete up-and-down counts as 1.

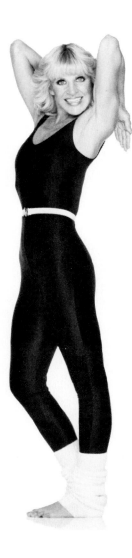

2A

Now put both elbows up and close to the ears (legs straight and together, or optionally bent if you want) and . . .

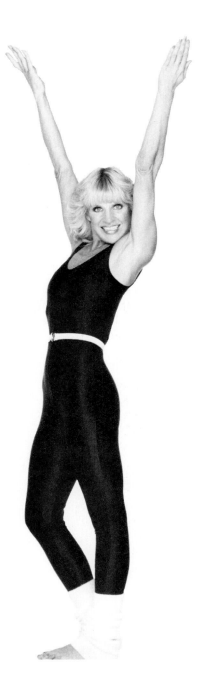

2B

. . . fling the arms straight up, keeping the elbows *glued* to the ears. Do 2 sets of 8.

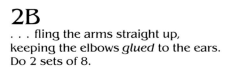

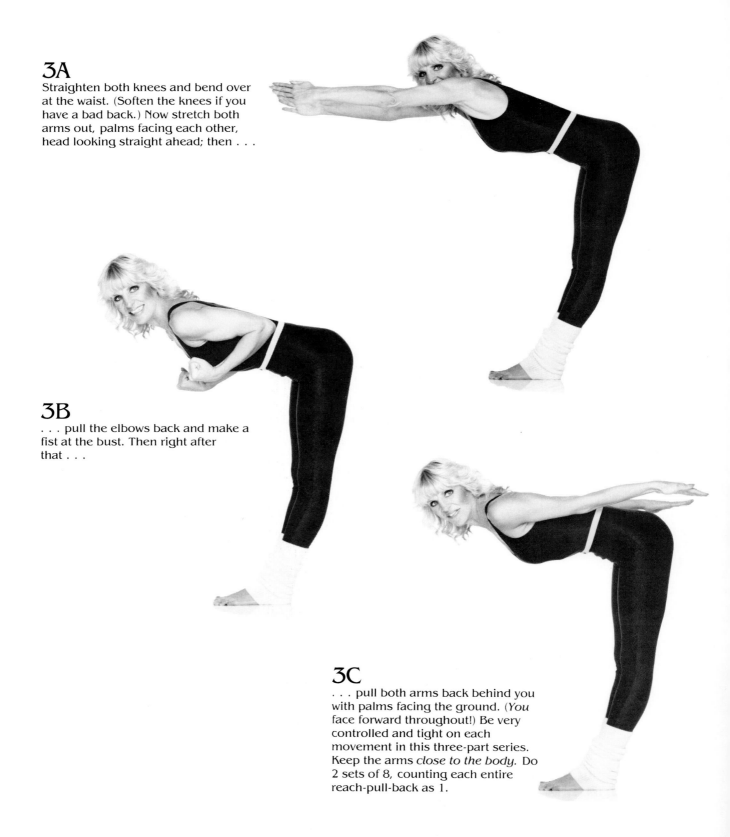

3A

Straighten both knees and bend over at the waist. (Soften the knees if you have a bad back.) Now stretch both arms out, palms facing each other, head looking straight ahead; then . . .

3B

. . . pull the elbows back and make a fist at the bust. Then right after that . . .

3C

. . . pull both arms back behind you with palms facing the ground. (*You face forward throughout!*) Be very controlled and tight on each movement in this three-part series. Keep the arms *close to the body.* Do 2 sets of 8, counting each entire reach-pull-back as 1.

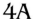

4A

Now for the reverse push-up. It's hard! Get into position as shown and . . .

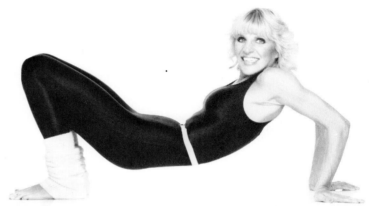

4B

. . . lower yourself by *bending the elbows* for 1 set of 8. If your back isn't strong, don't lift the body too high.

REPEAT

Go back to position 1 and repeat the entire routine. Keep going until your 5 minutes are up.

Thighs—5 Minutes

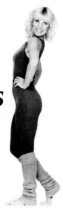

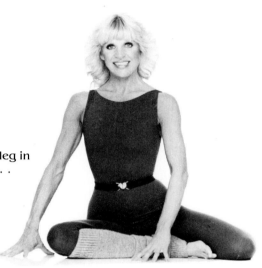

1A
Sit on the floor, legs bent, right leg in front and left leg behind, then . . .

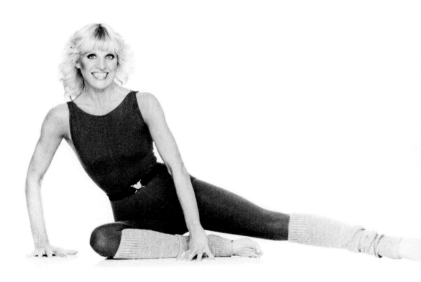

1B
. . . lift and lower the left leg at an angle. *Don't* let it touch either the other foot or the floor. Keep it up. Do 2 sets of 8.

2A
Now take that left leg and extend it with toe pointed. Then . . .

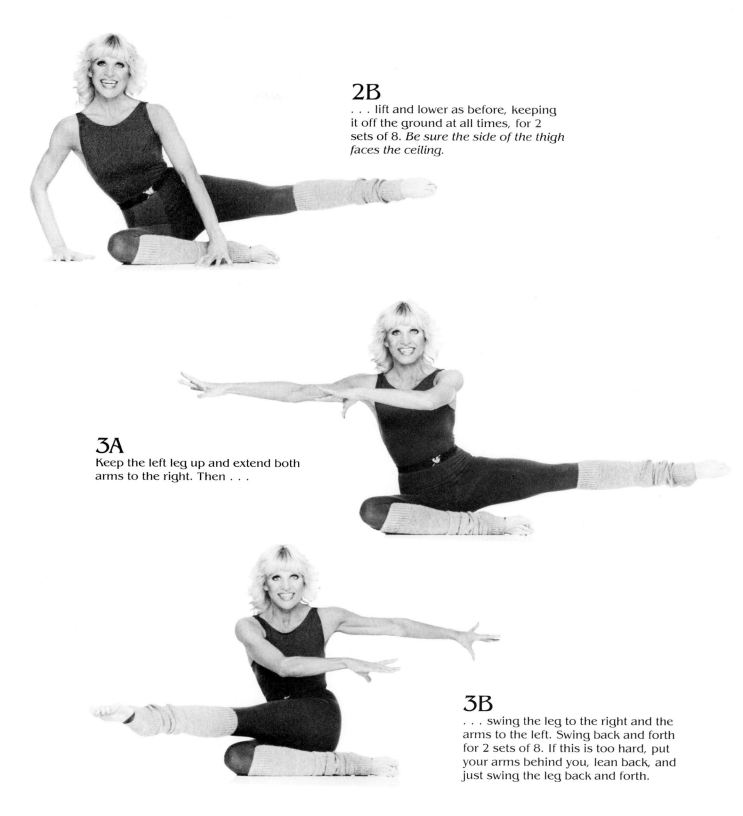

2B
. . . lift and lower as before, keeping it off the ground at all times, for 2 sets of 8. *Be sure the side of the thigh faces the ceiling.*

3A
Keep the left leg up and extend both arms to the right. Then . . .

3B
. . . swing the leg to the right and the arms to the left. Swing back and forth for 2 sets of 8. If this is too hard, put your arms behind you, lean back, and just swing the leg back and forth.

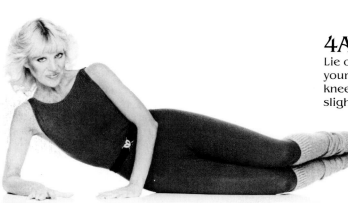

4A

Lie on your right side propped on your right elbow. Bend the legs at the knees and keep the feet together and slightly off the floor. Then . . .

4B

. . . open and shut the knees, keeping the toes together, for 1 set of 8.

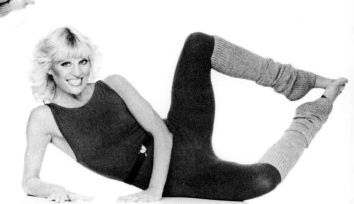

REPEAT

Go back to position 1A and repeat the entire routine on the other side. Keep going until your 5 minutes are up.

Feet Beat?

This'll make 'em really glamorous.

1. Soak feet in warm water, then smooth calluses with a pumice stone.
2. Apply a mask of chilled plain yogurt to both feet, leave on for 5 minutes, and rinse.
3. Cut nails short and straight across.
4. Apply opalescent nail polish.
5. Use a little gold-flecked powder on toes and heels.

Now they're irresistible.

Hips—5 Minutes

1A

Lie on your back, hands behind your head, legs bent, left ankle on right knee. Hold the stomach tight and . . .

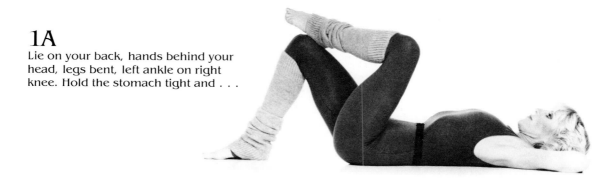

1B

. . . pulse up and squeeze the bottom for 2 sets of 8.

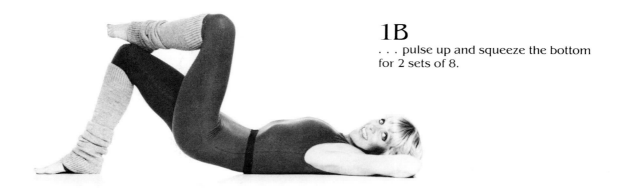

2A
This time extend the left leg straight up, toe pointed, and . . .

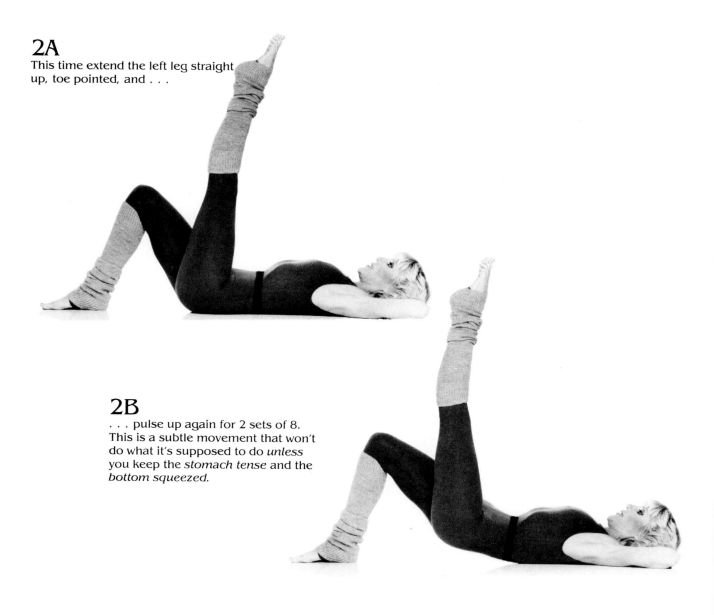

2B
. . . pulse up again for 2 sets of 8. This is a subtle movement that won't do what it's supposed to do *unless* you keep the *stomach tense* and the *bottom squeezed*.

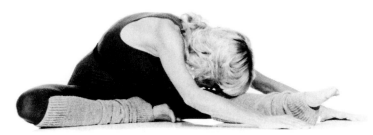

3A
Sit up, right leg folded, left leg extended, left toe pointed. Reach out both arms and bring your head down to your knee (or as close as possible), then . . .

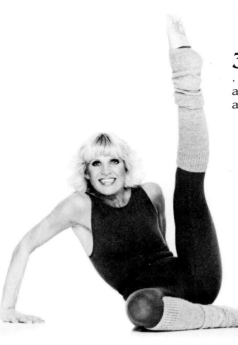

3B

. . . sit back, bringing the hands back and the left leg straight up. Go back and forth like this for 2 sets of 8.

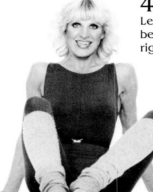

4A

Lean back on both hands, knees bent, left toe touching the top of the right foot. Then . . .

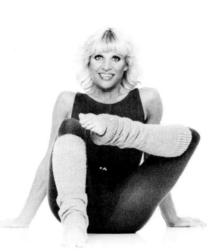

4B

. . . lift and lower the left foot so that the inner thigh of your left leg faces upward. Do 2 sets of 8.

REPEAT

Go back to position 1A and repeat the entire routine with the other leg, and go back and forth until your 5 minutes are up.

Bottom—5 Minutes

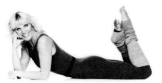

1

Lie on your stomach, head tucked down either on or alongside folded arms. Raise the left leg, foot pointed, off the ground and hold it there. Don't lift it so high that you feel *any* pain in the back. Now pulse the foot up another 12 inches and back, *not* letting it down to the floor, but always keeping it up in the air. Do 2 sets of 8.

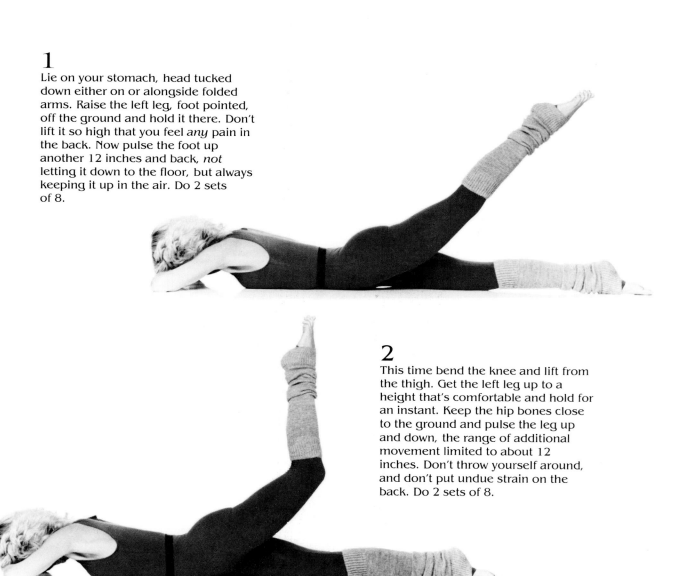

2

This time bend the knee and lift from the thigh. Get the left leg up to a height that's comfortable and hold for an instant. Keep the hip bones close to the ground and pulse the leg up and down, the range of additional movement limited to about 12 inches. Don't throw yourself around, and don't put undue strain on the back. Do 2 sets of 8.

3

Repeat position 1 with the other leg.

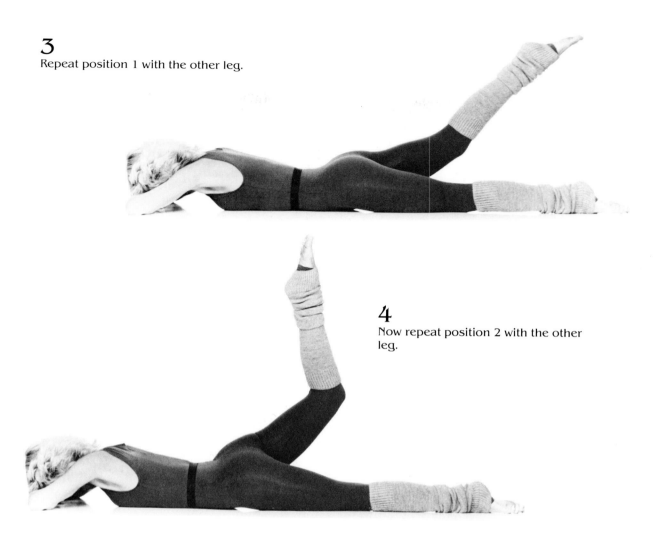

4

Now repeat position 2 with the other leg.

5A

Here's a tough one. Put the chin on the ground and the palms on your hips or upper thighs. Get as comfortable as you can and . . .

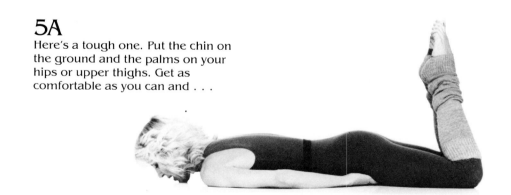

5B

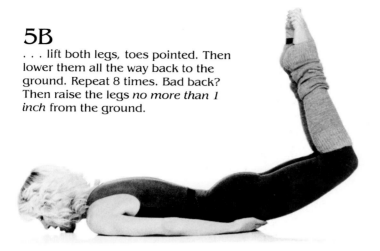

. . . lift both legs, toes pointed. Then lower them all the way back to the ground. Repeat 8 times. Bad back? Then raise the legs *no more than 1 inch* from the ground.

REPEAT

Go back to position 1 and repeat the entire routine. Keep going until your 5 minutes are up.

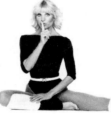

Cool-down—5 Minutes

Turn to pages 64–65 for your Total Shape-up II cool-down. Remember, no pulsing.

END OF TODAY'S TONING ROUTINES BYE-BYE!

Getting Fat Without Gaining Weight

Every year after the age of 35, the fat content of the normal human body increases by 1%. You don't even have to gain weight. Your body's fat content will inexorably grow all by itself. All the more reason to keep your muscles in shape.

Fascinating Fact

Exercise suppresses appetite—but only temporarily. As long as you're engaged in vigorous activity, both the blood circulation to the stomach and the resultant desire for food will be simultaneously reduced. However, things soon return to normal after you've finished your workout.

Calories and Exercise

Excess calories burned by virtue of exercise *don't* all come off while you're moving around. To the contrary, the bulk of these calories burn away during a 15-hour period *following* vigorous exercise.

Eating More

Since muscle requires more calories for maintenance than fat, if you're in good shape you can eat more and not gain weight.

When to Eat

An exercise session less than two hours after a meal interferes with digestion. But an apple, pear, or similar piece of fresh fruit *no less* than 30 minutes before exercise will give you additional energy for your workout.

Total
Shape-up III

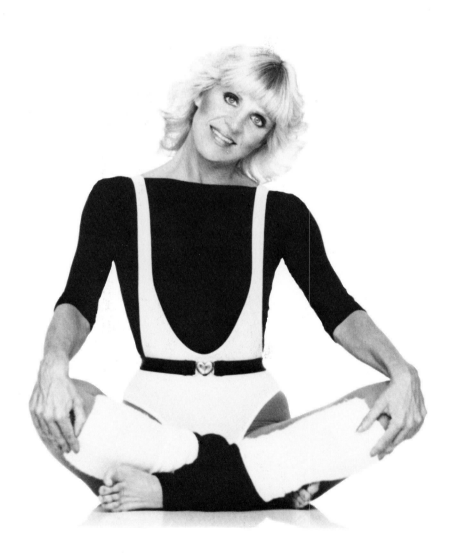

Total Shape-up III
Aerobic Routines for Monday, Wednesday, and Friday

Warm-up—5 Minutes

I hope you gave yourself a really wonderful present after finishing Total Shape-up II. You must be almost a pro, so let's get on with your Total Shape-up III warm-up.

1A
Sit cross-legged with the hands on the knees. Slowly and softly *pulse* the head first to the left . . .

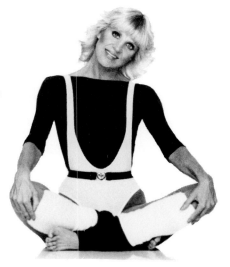

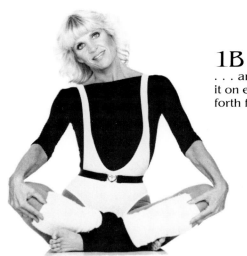

1B
. . . and then to the right. Don't hold it on either side, but pulse back and forth for a slow count of 10.

2A
Pull the knees out a little so that the soles of the feet touch. Clasp the feet with the hands and . . .

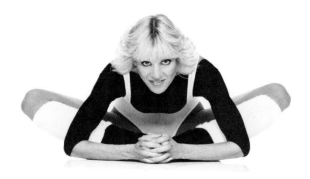

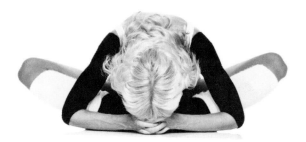

2B
. . . pulse forward, head down, for another slow count of 10. This stretches the inner thighs to counteract the drapery effect.

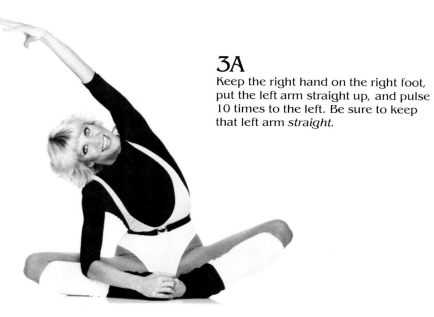

3A

Keep the right hand on the right foot, put the left arm straight up, and pulse 10 times to the left. Be sure to keep that left arm *straight*.

3B

Switch arms and do the same thing to the right, for another slow count of 10.

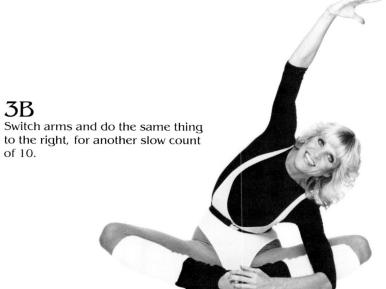

4A

Now spread the legs wide, point the toes, reach up with both arms, and . . .

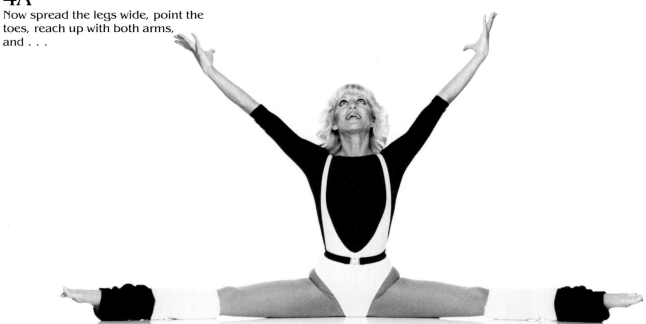

4B

. . . *lean forward at the waist,* arms outstretched. Do 10 slow dips, up and down. Keep the *bottom on the floor;* don't let it come up. And keep the chin *high.*

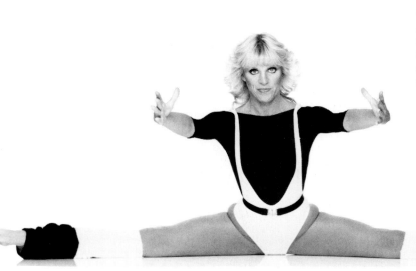

5A

Keep the legs in the same position, put your hands on the floor in front of you, and try to pulse yourself down as far as you can for a slow count of 10.

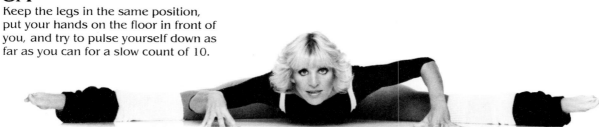

5B

And if you can come *all* the way down and grasp both ankles, then you should star in an exercise show of your own!

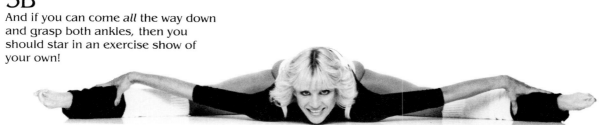

REPEAT

Go back to position 1A and repeat the entire routine. Keep going until your 5 minutes are up.

Staying Slim Is Easier for Men

Don't we women know it too. First there's menstruation, which leads to periodic weight-inducing hormone imbalances and water retention. Then there's the fact that we have 20% *more* fat cells in our bodies than men have in theirs. Not fair. Neither is the fact that muscle tissue requires more calorie-burning energy than fat. Therefore, since men are more muscular they *automatically* burn off more calories and lose weight faster than we do. Faced with these inequities all a woman can do is . . . work harder.

PUT ON YOUR SHOES
It's time for Aerobics—20 Minutes

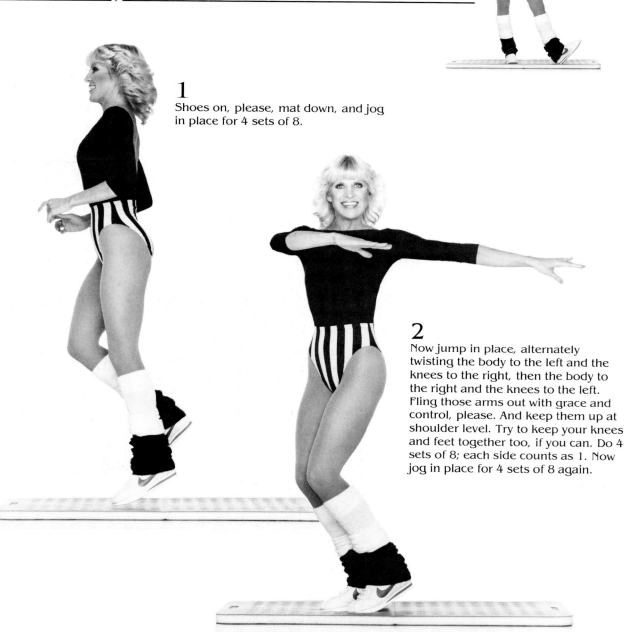

1
Shoes on, please, mat down, and jog in place for 4 sets of 8.

2
Now jump in place, alternately twisting the body to the left and the knees to the right, then the body to the right and the knees to the left. Fling those arms out with grace and control, please. And keep them up at shoulder level. Try to keep your knees and feet together too, if you can. Do 4 sets of 8; each side counts as 1. Now jog in place for 4 sets of 8 again.

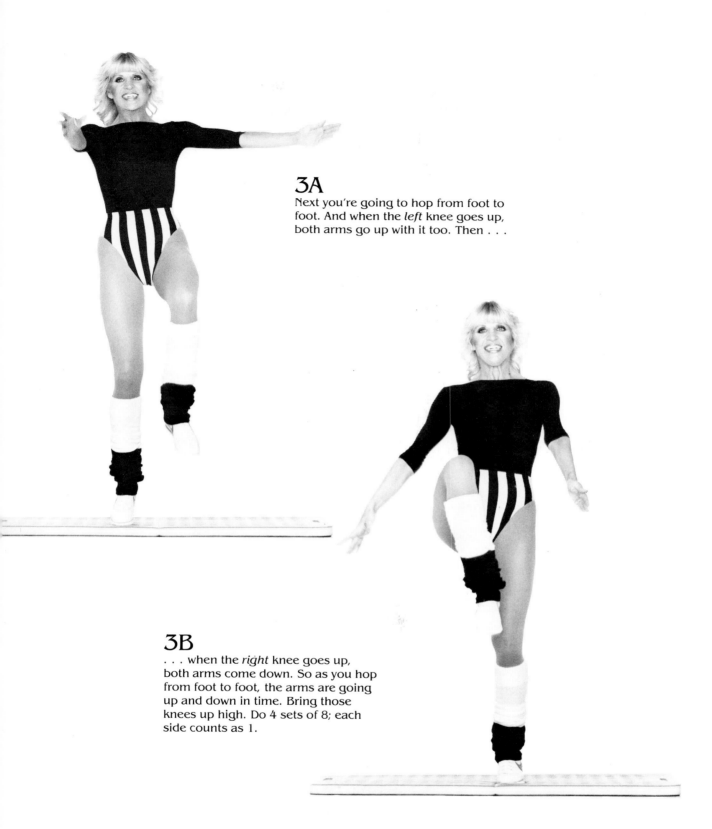

3A

Next you're going to hop from foot to foot. And when the *left* knee goes up, both arms go up with it too. Then . . .

3B

. . . when the *right* knee goes up, both arms come down. So as you hop from foot to foot, the arms are going up and down in time. Bring those knees up high. Do 4 sets of 8; each side counts as 1.

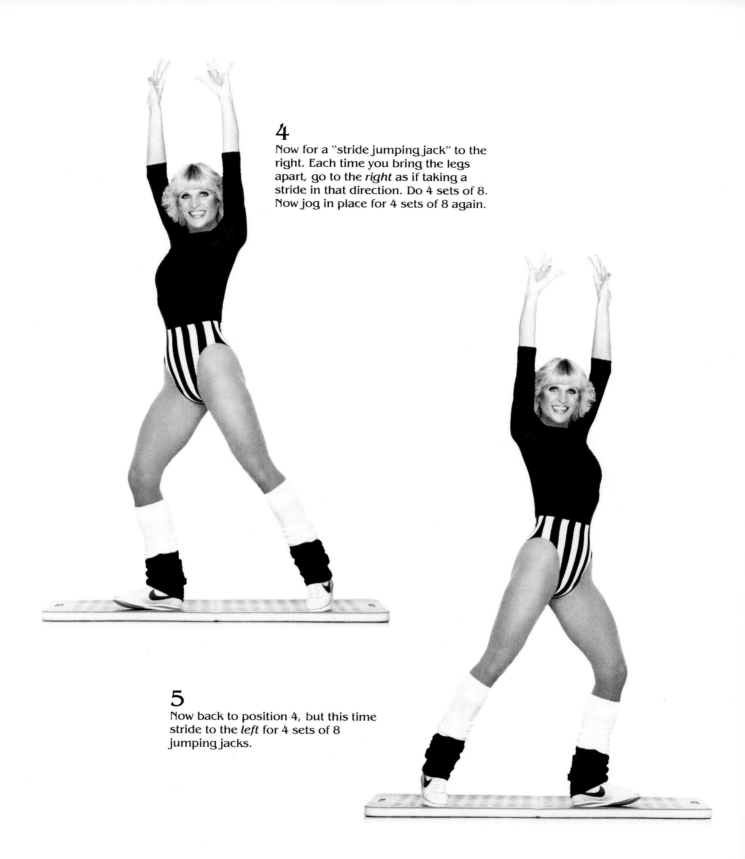

4

Now for a "stride jumping jack" to the right. Each time you bring the legs apart, go to the *right* as if taking a stride in that direction. Do 4 sets of 8. Now jog in place for 4 sets of 8 again.

5

Now back to position 4, but this time stride to the *left* for 4 sets of 8 jumping jacks.

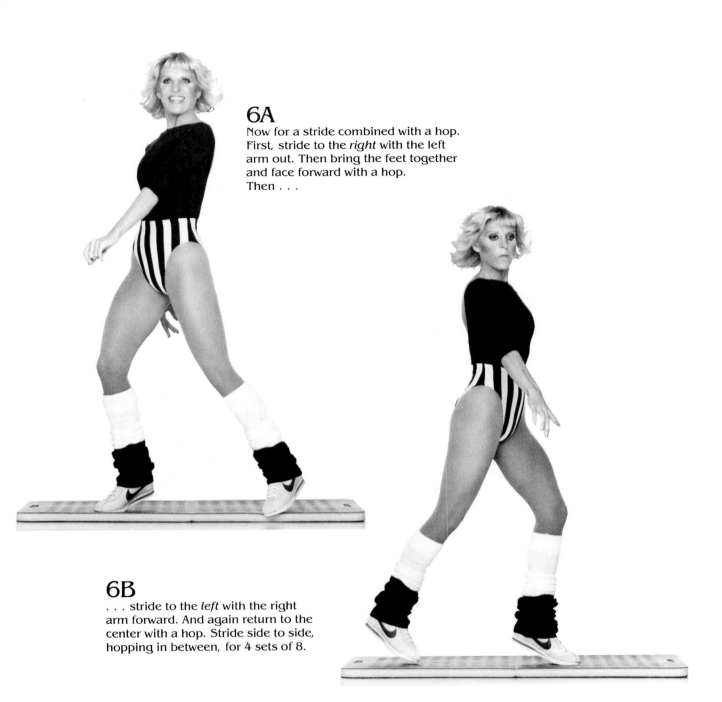

6A

Now for a stride combined with a hop. First, stride to the *right* with the left arm out. Then bring the feet together and face forward with a hop. Then . . .

6B

. . . stride to the *left* with the right arm forward. And again return to the center with a hop. Stride side to side, hopping in between, for 4 sets of 8.

REPEAT

Go back to position 1 and repeat the entire routine. Keep going until your 20 minutes are up.

Cellulite Is Nothing but Fat

The word (by the way, it rhymes with "parakeet") has become part of the language and can't be ignored. And as a matter of fact, most women *do* have thick layers of fat on their bottoms and thighs. And that fat *does* become dimpled and *is* hard to remove. But that doesn't make it anything other than fat.

A pound of fat results from 3,500 excess calories of *anything*. You eat it; you'll gain it. There's nothing exotic about it. Like all fat it responds eventually to plain old exercise and diet.

Don't Ask Dracula

What could help relieve the symptoms of: arthritis, hypertension, diabetes, pneumonia, anemia, infections, and meningitis?

Answer: *garlic*. It's no substitute for other medicines, of course, nor should it be taken in large quantities lest it upset your stomach and make your breath into a lethal weapon. But it does help.

The Ginger Cure

For airsickness eat ginger. *Not* gingersnaps, but ginger in capsule or powdered form. It really works and won't cause drowsiness.

Cool-down—5 Minutes

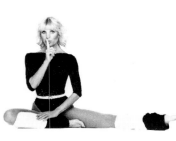

Easy music now. Forgo the driving beat. You've earned a rest.

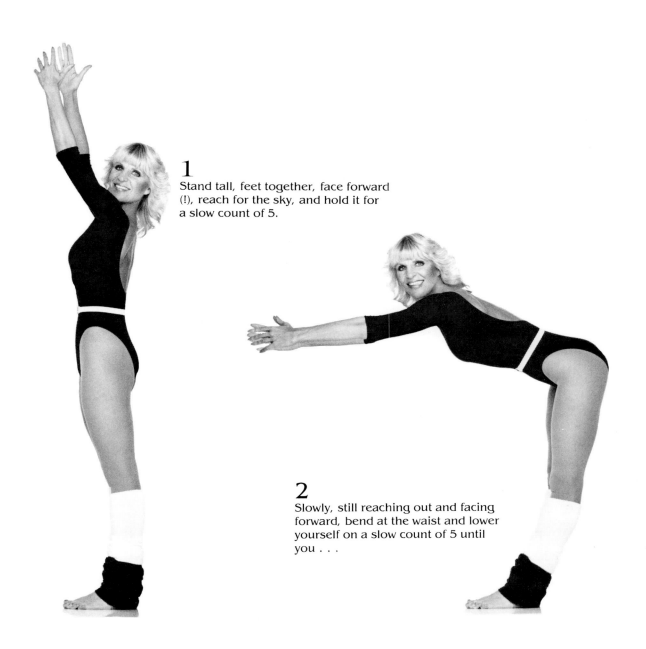

1
Stand tall, feet together, face forward (!), reach for the sky, and hold it for a slow count of 5.

2
Slowly, still reaching out and facing forward, bend at the waist and lower yourself on a slow count of 5 until you . . .

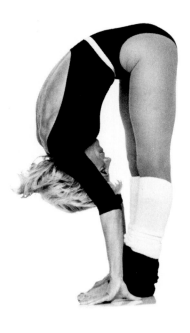

3

. . . touch your toes (or whatever you *can* touch). Now stay just like this for another slow count of 5.

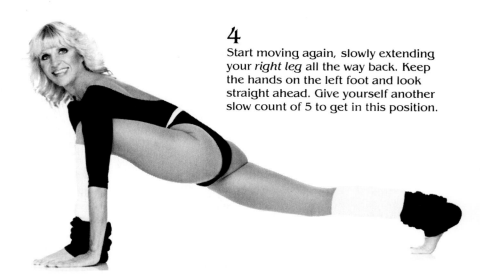

4

Start moving again, slowly extending your *right leg* all the way back. Keep the hands on the left foot and look straight ahead. Give yourself another slow count of 5 to get in this position.

5

Now then, over the next slow count to 5, I want you to bring the forward foot *back* to meet the other one, while at the same time you slowly lift your bottom up and bend at the waist.

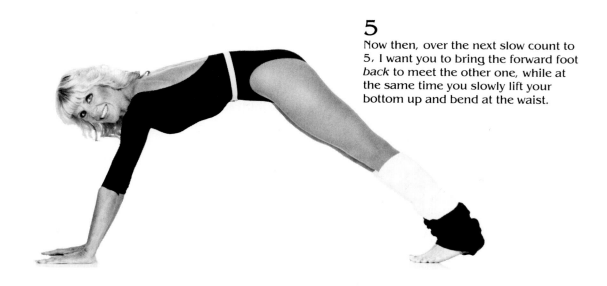

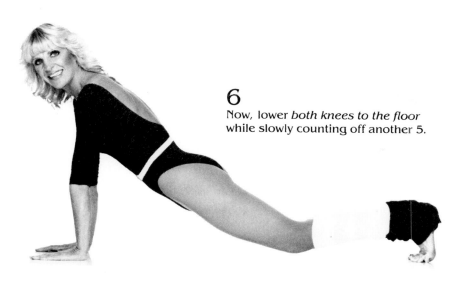

6

Now, lower *both knees to the floor* while slowly counting off another 5.

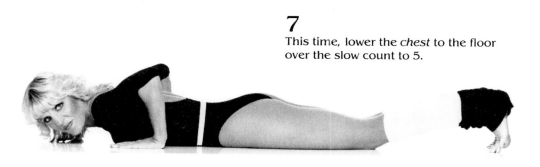

7

This time, lower the *chest* to the floor over the slow count to 5.

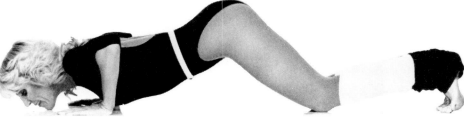

8

Push the bottom up, knees on the floor, back *arched,* in a sort of gradual modified push-up. At the end of another slow count of 5 you should be in . . .

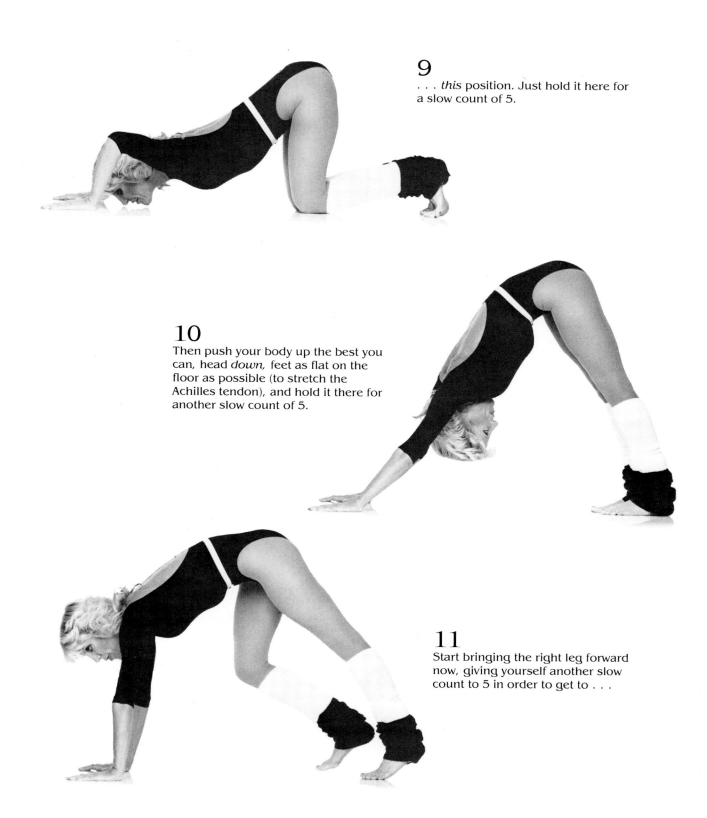

9

. . . *this* position. Just hold it here for a slow count of 5.

10

Then push your body up the best you can, head *down,* feet as flat on the floor as possible (to stretch the Achilles tendon), and hold it there for another slow count of 5.

11

Start bringing the right leg forward now, giving yourself another slow count to 5 in order to get to . . .

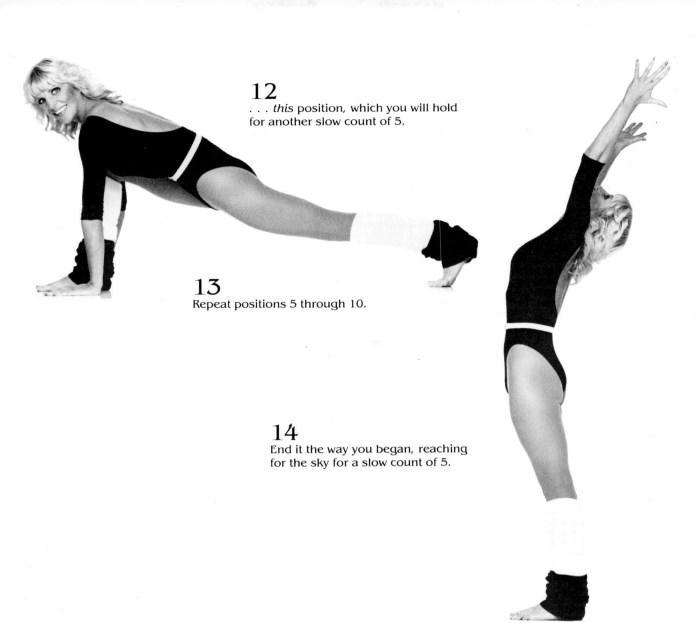

12
. . . *this* position, which you will hold for another slow count of 5.

13
Repeat positions 5 through 10.

14
End it the way you began, reaching for the sky for a slow count of 5.

REPEAT

Go back to position 1 and repeat the entire routine. Keep going until your 5 minutes are up.

END OF TODAY'S AEROBIC ROUTINES
BYE-BYE!

What's Good for Ulcers?

Since ancient times people have used licorice for digestive problems. Of course, too much is a bad thing. But used in moderation it's very soothing.

Nature's Remedy for Indigestion

Dried slices of papaya are great for upset stomachs. The reason: Papaya contains papain, a protein-digesting enzyme.

Cold Milk at Bedtime

Milk contains L-tryptophan, a substance that helps put you to sleep. However, heating the milk *depletes* the L-tryptophan, thereby making it less likely to make you sleepy! Although warm milk tastes great at bedtime, if you need help falling asleep you'd better drink it cold.

Total Shape-up III

Toning Routines for Tuesday and Thursday

Warm-up—5 Minutes

Turn to the instructions on pages 95–99 for your Total Shape-up III pre-toning warm-up. And remember to *breathe!*

De-tense Fast

Here's a quick maneuver when you're tired at the end of the day but have to keep going.

Take off your shoes, wiggle your toes, run the soles of your feet over the rung of a chair.

Sit quietly and turn your head slowly and evenly from side to side. Let the head drop toward first one shoulder, then the other.

Keeping the head relaxed and erect, hold the skin at the back of the neck and squeeze and let go several times. Do the same to the shoulders.

Finally, put your fingers atop the tender spots on your neck and shoulders and press with a circular motion.

Waist—5 Minutes

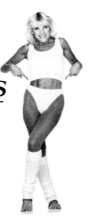

1

Here's your position: Fold your left leg back (*don't* sit on your foot); fold your right leg in front; lace the fingers behind the head.

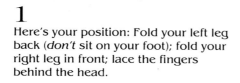

2

Tilt to the left, keeping the *hips on the ground.* Pulse (don't jerk) for 1 set of 8.

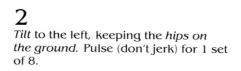

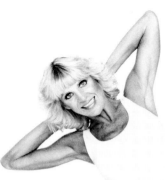

3

Now tilt to the opposite side for another set of 8.

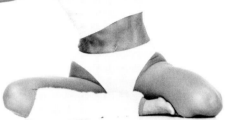

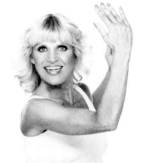

4A

Cross both legs in front of you Tonto-style, hold the palms up, elbows at *shoulder level,* and do a *double pulse* to the *left.* Twist your body, but keep the head facing *forward.* After your double pulse to the left . . .

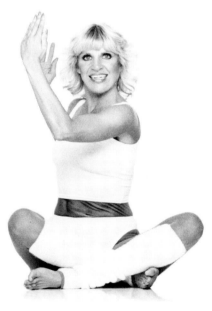

4B

. . . come around and do a double pulse to the right. Alternate left and right for 1 set of 8.

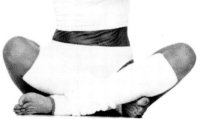

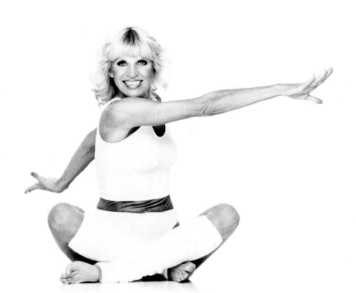

5A

Stay in the same position, and do the same alternate double pulses, but this time fling the right arm forward and the left arm back when you pulse to the left . . .

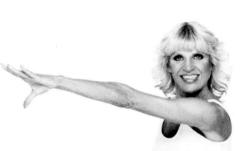

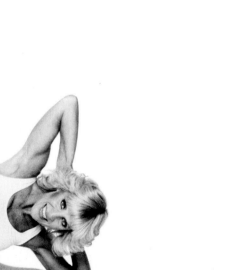

5B

. . . and switch the arms the other way when you pulse to the right. Do 1 set of 8; each side counts as 1.

6A

Spread the legs apart, point the toes, lace the hands behind the head, and do a *single pulse,* first to the left . . .

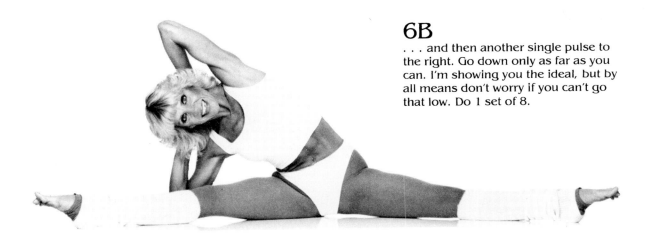

6B

. . . and then another single pulse to the right. Go down only as far as you can. I'm showing you the ideal, but by all means don't worry if you can't go that low. Do 1 set of 8.

7A

Finally, touch the opposite toes windmill-style, first the left toe with the right hand . . .

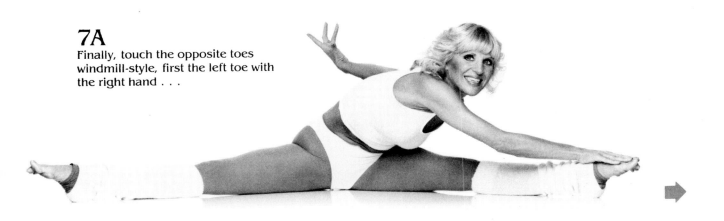

7B

. . . then the right toe with the left
hand. Do 1 set of 8.

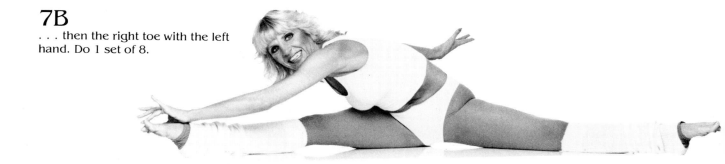

REPEAT

Go back to position 1 and repeat the entire waist routine.
Keep going until your 5 minutes are up.

You Don't Knead It

A good masseuse can be very effective at
breaking up and moving around deposits of
body fat. But *you've* got to burn the fat off yourself; no masseuse can do that for you.

The same goes for exotic "body wraps." They
may draw out excess water, but they don't af-
fect levels of fat. Only diet and exercise get rid
of that.

Stomach—5 Minutes

1

Sit on the floor, body *leaning* backward, face forward, arms extended parallel to the floor, palms facing up. Instead of lying all the way back, pulse the body up and down for 1 set of 8. By the way, this and the next exercise are both aimed at the midriff.

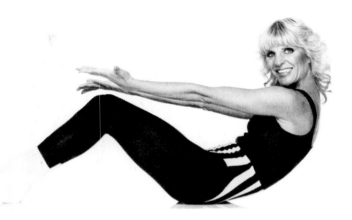

2A

Now put your hands on your knees and keep the body at a backward tilt. *Hold that stomach in!* Then . . .

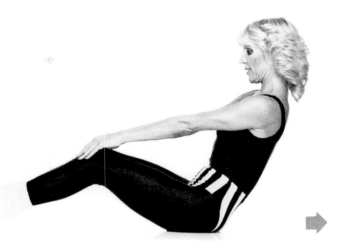

2B
. . . reach way around to the left, following your hand with your face . . .

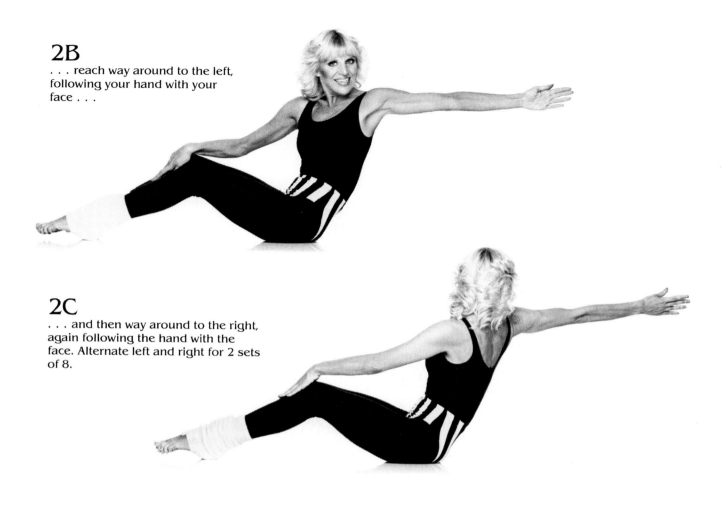

2C
. . . and then way around to the right, again following the hand with the face. Alternate left and right for 2 sets of 8.

3A
For the potbelly we're going to put both hands behind the back, pull the knees up to the face, point the toes (face forward of course), and . . .

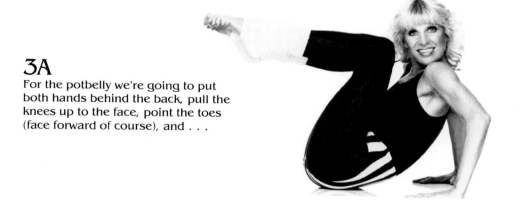

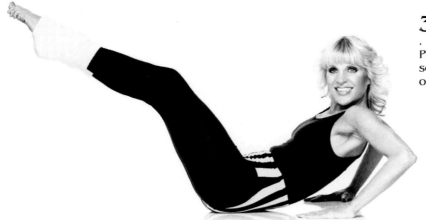

3B

. . . push the legs out and slightly up. Pretend you're a clothespin being squeezed open and shut for 1 set of 8.

4A

For the obliques and the transverses you're going to do essentially the same motion. But this time extend the legs . . .

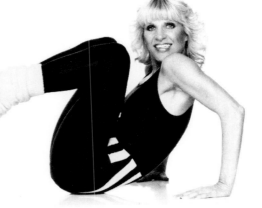

4B

. . . on a *diagonal,* first to the left, and then . . .

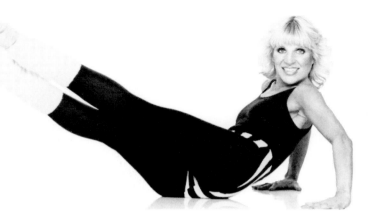

4C

. . . on a *diagonal* to the right. Do 1 set of 8.

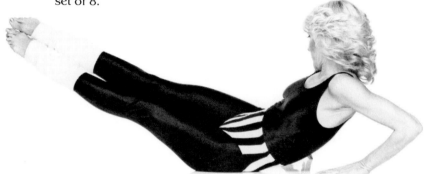

REPEAT

Go back to position 1 and repeat the entire routine. Keep going until your 5 minutes are up.

Arms and Pectorals (Bust)—
5 Minutes

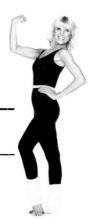

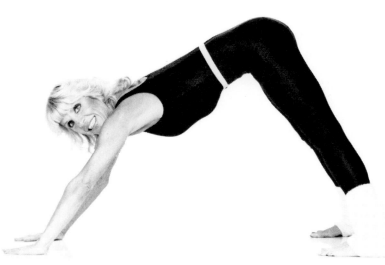

1A
Stand on all fours with your hands and feet not too close together, keep the legs apart and the heels down (if possible), then . . .

1B
. . . bend the arms push-up fashion and touch the forehead to the floor. Keep the back *straight.* Do 2 sets of 8, or the most you can.

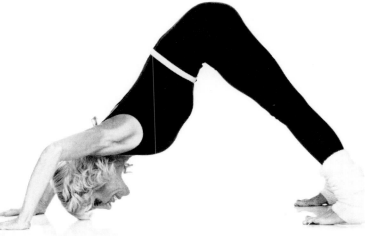

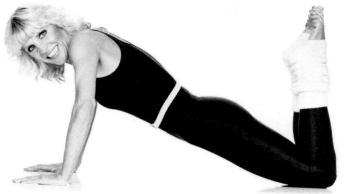

2A

This is your basic bent-leg push-up. If you can't bend your knees like this, just keep the legs straight and . . .

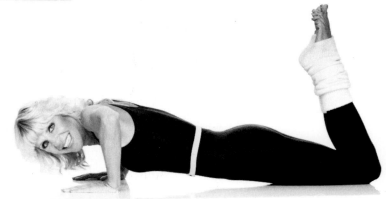

2B

. . . lower and raise yourself in push-up style for 2 sets of 8.

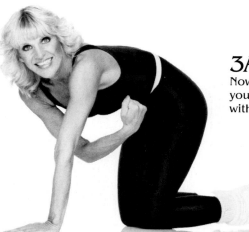

3A

Now for the underarm fling. Get on your hands and knees, make a fist with the right hand, and . . .

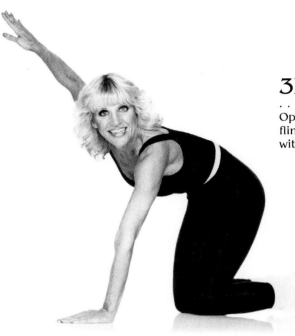

3B

. . . fling it out and up to the side. Open your fingers on the upward fling, and follow your moving hand with your face. Do 2 sets of 8.

4

Now do another 2 sets of 8 underarm flings with the other arm.

5A

Sit cross-legged, elbows *close to the ears,* face forward, palms *on the back.*

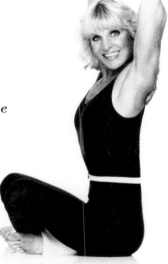

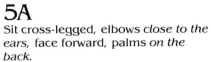

5B
Extend the right hand up as shown, then bring it back down.

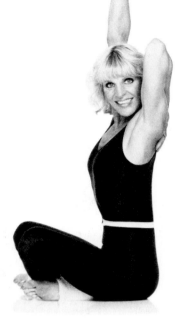

5C
Then extend the left hand the same way, and bring it back too. Alternate hands, patting yourself on the back each time, for 2 sets of 8.

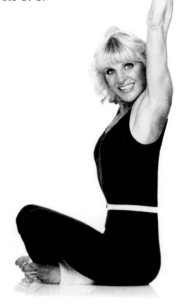

REPEAT

Go back to position 1A and repeat the entire routine. Keep going until your 5 minutes are up.

"Space Invader" Face Lifts

Have you heard about the new nonsurgical way to tighten sagging faces with helium laser beams? Why, it sounds too good to be true. That's because it *is* too good to be true.

Laser face lifts are highlighted by theatrical red lighting and a healing sensation of warmth. The heat produced during treatment may indeed temporarily smooth facial tissue by means of minor swelling. But there is no evidence the treatment produces any *permanent* positive effect at all.

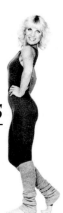

Thighs—5 Minutes

1

Assume the Standard Poodle hydrant position, *left* leg up and bent at the knee. Point the toe and be *sure* the outer thigh faces the ceiling. Distribute your weight evenly on both hands and *try not to lean*. Now, do a mini-lift with the left leg, keeping it aloft at all times and pulsing it up and down. Do 2 sets of 8.

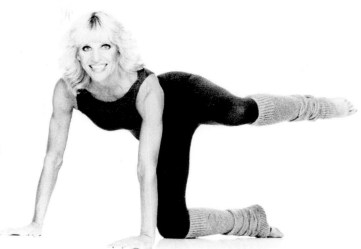

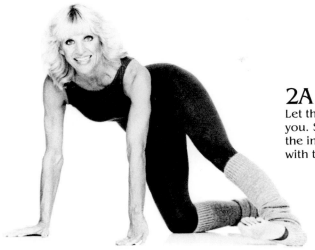

2A

Let the left leg down a bit in front of you. Straighten the knee and place the instep on the floor. Flex the foot with toes pulled back and . . .

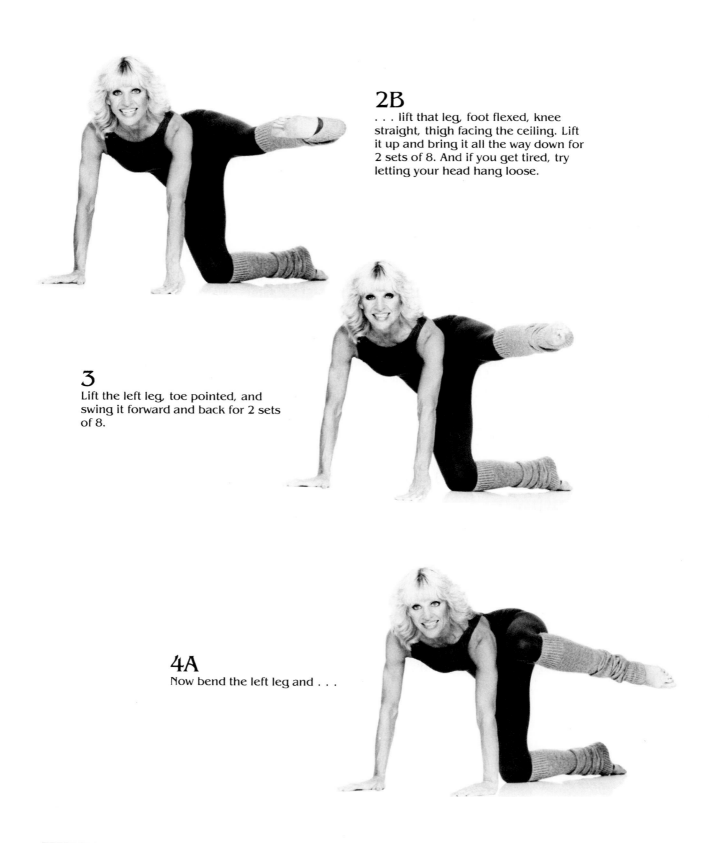

2B

. . . lift that leg, foot flexed, knee straight, thigh facing the ceiling. Lift it up and bring it all the way down for 2 sets of 8. And if you get tired, try letting your head hang loose.

3

Lift the left leg, toe pointed, and swing it forward and back for 2 sets of 8.

4A

Now bend the left leg and . . .

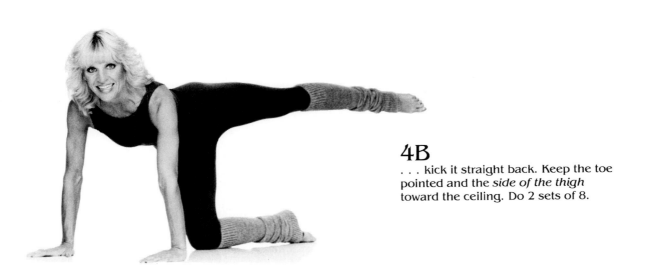

4B

. . . kick it straight back. Keep the toe pointed and the *side of the thigh* toward the ceiling. Do 2 sets of 8.

5A

Next, extend the left leg back, then . . .

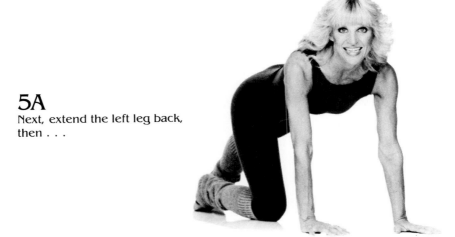

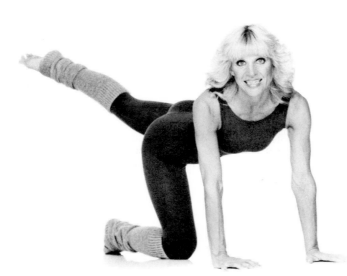

5B
. . . lift it up and over the right foot, and . . .

5C
. . . touch it to the floor. Go back and forth over the right foot for 2 sets of 8; each time the toe touches the ground counts as 1.

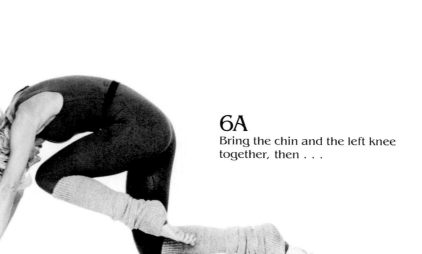

6A
Bring the chin and the left knee together, then . . .

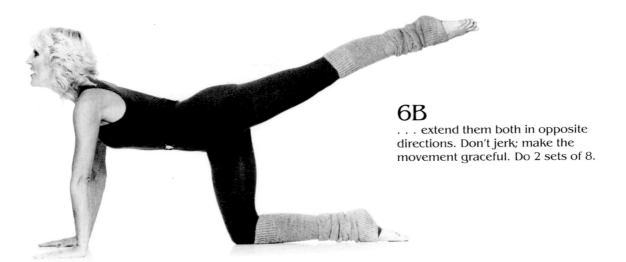

6B

. . . extend them both in opposite directions. Don't jerk; make the movement graceful. Do 2 sets of 8.

REPEAT

Go back to position 1 and repeat the entire routine with the other leg. Keep going until your 5 minutes are up.

Nixing Knee Pains

Knee problems plague women much more than they do men. This is thought to be because of the greater width of the female pelvis, which puts additional stress on the female knee.

Knee problems can be avoided almost entirely if proper attention is given to *warm-ups* and *leg exercises.*

The wrong shoes contribute to knee pains too. If you jump rope, you need a cushioned flat-soled shoe. If you run, you need a shoe with a raised heel.

Hips—5 Minutes

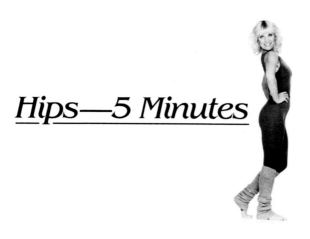

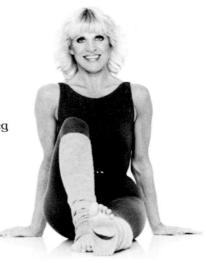

1A
Sit and smile, right knee bent, left leg extended, foot pointed. Then . . .

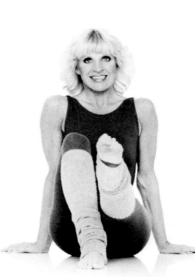

1B
. . . raise and lower the left leg for 2 sets of 8, and *don't let it touch the floor!*

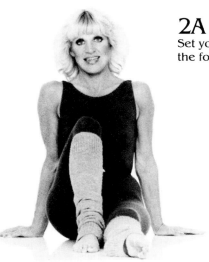

2A

Set your leg down for a moment, turn the foot out, keep it pointed, and . . .

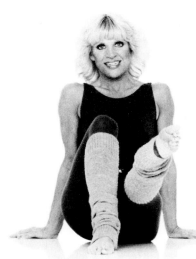

2B

. . . lift it up and down again for another 2 sets of 8. Be sure that it doesn't touch the floor and that you keep it pointed and turned out.

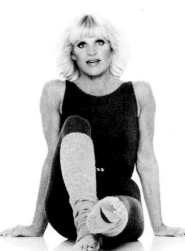

3A

Keep that left foot pointed still, and turned out, and off the ground, and . . .

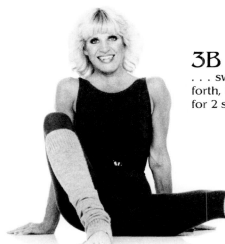

3B

. . . swing it to the side. Go back and forth, keeping the leg off the ground, for 2 sets of 8.

4A

Now for the hip roll—which looks harder than it really is. All you do is roll on the hips first to the left, then to the right. Keep the feet off the ground if you can; if not don't panic. When you're on the left hip raise the right hand, and . . .

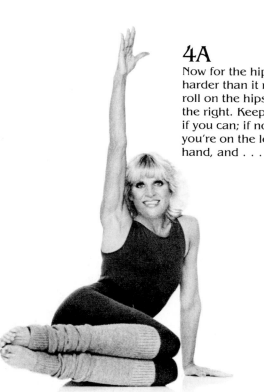

4B

. . . when you're on the right hip, raise the left hand. Go back and forth for 2 sets of 8.

REPEAT

Go back to position 1A and repeat the entire routine with the other leg, and repeat the hip roll at the end. Keep going until your 5 minutes are up. (Don't forget! When time is up, *finish the complete routine before moving on.*)

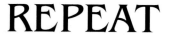

Bottom—5 Minutes

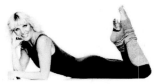

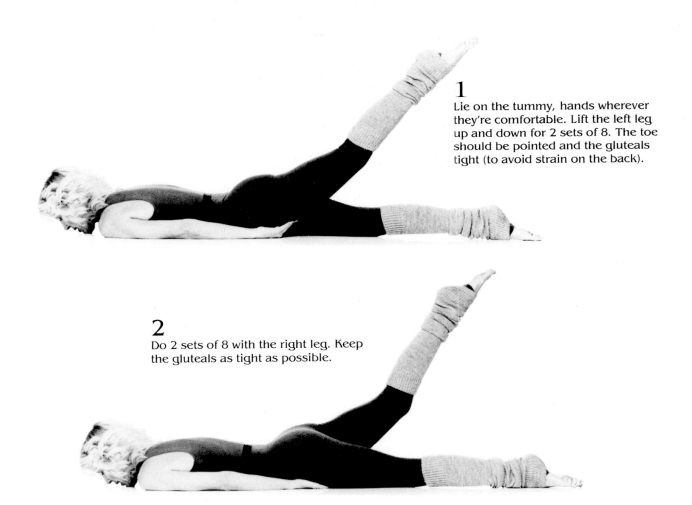

1

Lie on the tummy, hands wherever they're comfortable. Lift the left leg up and down for 2 sets of 8. The toe should be pointed and the gluteals tight (to avoid strain on the back).

2

Do 2 sets of 8 with the right leg. Keep the gluteals as tight as possible.

3

This time lift *both* legs for 2 sets of 8. They don't have to go very high. In fact, don't even try to get them high unless you're in extraordinary shape already. The main thing is to squeeze and be in control.

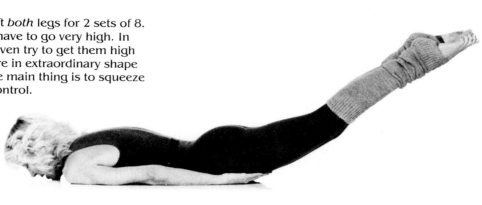

4A

Now spread the legs, toes pointed, and . . .

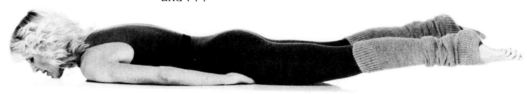

4B

. . . scissor back and forth, alternating feet over and under, for 2 sets of 8. And keep the gluteals tight.

REPEAT

Go back to position 1 and repeat the entire routine. Keep going until your 5 minutes are up.

Cool-down—5 Minutes

Follow the Total Shape-up III cool-down instructions on pages 105–109. Remember to hold your poses and *stretch*.

END OF TODAY'S TONING ROUTINES
BYE-BYE!

Twin Pickups for Tired Eyes

1. Press cotton balls dipped in witch hazel against your eyelids; or
2. Place mint leaves under your eyes and take a nap.

Five Common Vitamin Robbers

1. Oral contraceptives. They block efficient absorption of both Vitamin C and the B-complex vitamins. You should take a multivitamin supplement every day.
2. Tetracycline. The ubiquitous anti-acne medicine causes an unsuspected but significant excretion of Vitamin C. Take 500 milligrams daily to offset the effect. Many drugs impair vitamin absorption; ask your doctor if he's prescribed one for you.
3. Menstruation. Robs you of iron. A daily multivitamin *with iron* will put things right.
4. Vegetarianism: Those who don't eat meat don't get enough of the B12 vitamins contained so abundantly in meat and poultry. Rx: Take a daily supplement.
5. Smoking. If you do you're losing Vitamin C and need 500 milligrams a day in supplement form.

The Total Shape-up Diet—Tips That Trim

Do I really need to say anything in support of being slim? No heart likes laboring to pump blood around pounds and pounds of extra flesh. No muscle wants to strain itself needlessly to move flabby limbs and trunks. Big is *not* beautiful. Life is hard enough without adding effort to every move you make.

Before You Start

Here is a deceptively simple truth: People get fat by overeating, and they lose weight by cutting back. It's the rare individual who can lay the blame on "glands" or an aberrant metabolism. The normal person gets fat because he's pigging out.

I'm not very concerned about people who are 10 or maybe even 15 pounds too heavy, although they'd look better lighter. But carrying around more than 15 extra pounds is as bad for one's health as it is for one's agility and stamina.

How much should you weigh? If you're going on a diet you'll need a specific target, and the table below should help you determine it. Remember, people with slight builds and narrow frames should aim for the low end of the appropriate weight range; those with broader builds can afford to weigh in nearer the top limits and still look trim.

IDEAL WEIGHT RANGE FOR WOMEN
(Men: add 5 pounds)

Height	Ideal Weight
5′ -5′2″	95-110
5′2″ -5′4″	105-120
5′4″ -5′6″	110-130
5′6″ -5′8″	120-140
5′8″ -5′10″	125-145
5′10″-6′	140-160

When it comes to reaching your weight goal, however, there are few things as potentially disappointing as fad diets. Almost all of them rob you of energy, mislead you with false promises, and initiate (or prolong) an unhealthy yo-yo syndrome wherein you are alternately fat and thin, fat and thin, fat and thin. Most of the time you'll probably be fat, since no one can *live* on a fad diet for any length of time.

Here's why. Each person has his or her own "set point" or level of stored fat. It's the weight you naturally maintain—give or take a few pounds—when you eat normally, neither dieting nor over-eating. Your body balances caloric intake, metabolic efficiency, and physical activity to maintain this amount of fat. But it does so without regard to reserves of energy or physical beauty.

When a diet takes you below the set point, your body goes into revolt. It wants to get those fat levels back up to where they were pre-diet. And it usually succeeds, which is why dieting alone rarely achieves long-term results.

Exercise seems to have a direct impact on the set point. Studies have shown that people who start a regular exercise program get thinner and stay thinner. And the reason is thought to be that regular exercise lowers the set point.

To lose weight effectively and permanently once you've started exercising, there is, in my opinion, *one more sensible course of action required:* Learn to count calories. You'd be surprised to discover how many calories are contained in some of the things you love—and how few are contained in others.

To learn caloric values, go to a bookstore, drugstore, or super-market and buy a good calorie-counting book. *Calories and Car-bohydrates* by Barbara Kraus (a Plume Book published by New American Library) and *The Complete Calorie Counter* by Elaine Chaback (published by Dell) are two that I like. Take your book and look up *everything* you eat. *Count every single bite and sip.* After a while you'll remember caloric values the way you remember telephone numbers. And soon you'll be able to estimate those things that aren't even listed in your book. Note your calories throughout the day and total them by bedtime. If you go over your quota, consume fewer calories tomorrow.

You can determine how many calories you should consume each day with fair accuracy by the following formula: Find your ideal weight on the chart above and multiply it by 15. The result will closely approximate the maximum number of calories you can eat each day without exceeding that ideal weight.

Next you must decide how fast you want to lose your extra weight. If each day you consume that number of calories sufficient to sustain your *ideal* weight, then gradually but inevitably you will start to shed the extra pounds—until you arrive at your ideal level. It won't happen fast. But then slow weight loss is usually preferable to the rapid variety, since banished weight stays off longer and slow diets are less of an ordeal. If you want to lose your extra pounds quickly, my advice then is to *cut 10%* from whatever calorie quota is required to support your ideal weight.

My Diet Plan for You

The Total Shape-up Diet is based on the following principles. You may want to discuss them with your doctor before you get started. Basically, they are all about getting the most energy from the fewest calories.

• Frequently, I substitute grains, nuts, and seeds for meat, poultry, and dairy products. These are *all* sources of protein, but mine are less caloric and less liable to leave toxic residues in the tissues. I'm not telling you to become a vegetarian. But instead of eating meat three times a day why not have it just once?

• I try to select only fresh foods, because they have the most nutrients. The freezing process is great for convenience but not for food value.

• I avoid foods made with refined grains and sugar. Delicious as they often are, they seethe with empty calories. Besides, things made with coarse grains and whole wheat are much more nutritious.

• I try to eat and cook with as little animal fat as possible. OK, a little butter here and there won't hurt. But I use it sparingly and cook with vegetable oil instead.

• Overcooking destroys the natural nutritional value of food. The more *raw* food I eat the better I feel. About half my daily intake is completely uncooked.

• I eat only when I'm hungry. This may mean skipping a meal, but I'd rather do that than eat out of habit. Our bodies would naturally regulate the amount we eat, and thereby avoid overweight, if we didn't constantly override our instincts and eat because the clock says it's mealtime.

• Many small meals are better than few big ones. Spreading food intake evenly over the day counteracts occasional episodes of low blood sugar which rob us of energy and provoke eating sprees.

• I supplement my daily diet with a multivitamin. If I was positive of getting every single nutrient I needed I wouldn't bother. But I'm not. Between processing, preparation, cooking, and storage in the refrigerator, even the freshest foods will inevitably lose food value.

Particularly when you're dieting you run the risk of not getting all the vitamins you need. Vitamin supplements make everything easier. Can you imagine the amounts of food you'd have to eat to get enough Vitamin C to counteract stress, or Vitamin B to replenish what birth-control pills wash out of you? And so on down a long list.

Although most good multivitamins have virtually everything you need, I also take an extra supplement of Vitamin B12, since I'm a vegetarian and need it for energy.

Women who can't tolerate milk products should consider a calcium supplement too, say 800 milligrams a day.

• I drink *lots* of water. Four to six 8-ounce glasses each day will aid weight loss.

• Coffee and tea are OK, but herbal tea (chamomile, peppermint, etc.) is *always* to be preferred simply because it contains no caffeine.

• Wine and alcohol are OK too, but in moderation. Alcohol is fattening.

If you only took one single vitamin pill in your life, would you expect to know if it helped you? Or suppose you wonder whether or not jogging would improve your energy level. Would a single run be enough to tell? Of course not. You have to take vitamin pills for months to feel the difference. The same goes for jogging. And the same goes for my diet plan too. Here it is: day-to-day, meal-to-meal.

Give it at least two to four weeks. The foods are inexpensive, quick to prepare, and just as easy to order in restaurants.

Before breakfast: Have a glass of water into which you have squeezed the juice of either a lemon, a grapefruit, or an orange. Or have a cup of tea (herbal, please).

Breakfast: Make it light. Heavy breakfasts require too much energy to digest and can make you tired. Have tea plus one of the following: a piece of fresh fruit and a slice of cheese; a bowl of whole-grain cereal and skim milk; a slice of whole-grain bread spread with honey; or one of my "Good Morning Energizers."

Mid-morning snack: The point is to bolster flagging blood sugar levels, which *can* be accomplished without a hot fudge sundae. Have a piece of fresh fruit or a glass of vegetable juice.

The Florida Express

For instant go-power.

In a blender, combine

    1 cup low-fat milk

    2 heaping tablespoons of instant nonfat powdered milk

    2 heaping tablespoons of frozen orange juice concentrate

Blend just enough to mix.

Blast-off Supreme

One glass and you're ready for anything.

In a blender, combine:

¾ cup low-fat milk

¼ cup pitted prunes (about five small ones)

1 tablespoon unsulfured molasses (the unbitter one)

Blend until the prunes are thoroughly mixed up.

Tropical Sunrise

A more exotic taste.

Again in the blender, combine:

1 heaping tablespoon frozen apple juice concentrate

1 heaping tablespoon frozen orange juice concentrate

1 heaping tablespoon frozen pineapple juice concentrate

Ice cubes as needed

Add the ice cubes one by one to make the drink thick and frothy. Experiment to get the consistency you like.

"Morning After" Pickup

Here's an Rx for post-party drain. In a blender combine:

—8 ounces carrot juice

—4 ounces coconut milk

—3 400-milligram capsules of chlorella (a type of algae)

These are all health-food items, the purchase of which may require a special trip. But if you've got a big weekend coming up you're smart to have them on hand. The mixture is cooling, thirst-quenching, high in protein, and very restorative.

Lunch: There *are* alternatives to a cheeseburger deluxe, cheese-cake, and a chocolate malt. Have a plate of cottage cheese with fruit; a bowl of vegetable soup with greens; a plate of fresh fruit, raw vegetables, and nuts; or one of my "Lunches with Punches" as a main course.

Swiss Reuben

Very satisfying and surprisingly lo-cal.

1 slice of bread (of choice)
Dijon mustard (preferably)
Sauerkraut
2 slices Swiss cheese

Spread the bread with mustard, cover with warmed and well-drained sauerkraut, and top with the slices of Swiss cheese. Put in the broiler (about 4 inches from the heat) until bubbly.

Cheese Surprise

Guaranteed to convert cottage cheese haters.

¼ cup cottage cheese
2 tablespoons grated Parmesan cheese
Seeds (sesame, poppy, or caraway)
1 thick tomato slice
1 slice bread (of choice)

Mix the cottage cheese and grated Parmesan, and sprinkle with seeds of choice. Toast the bread, lay on the tomato slice, and top with the cheese mixture. At this point, either eat as is, or pop in the broiler (again about 4 inches from the heat) until bubbly.

Tom Sauce's Pizza

Mamma mia!

1 slice bread (of choice)
Tomato sauce
Oregano or basil
2 slices mozzarella cheese

Toast the bread and spread with tomato sauce. Sprinkle with a little oregano or basil, then layer with the two slices of cheese. Pop it in the broiler, 4 inches from the heat, until bubbly.

Saladorama

The crazy mixed-up salad.

2 heaping tablespoons plain yogurt
A little fresh dill
Shredded cabbage
Torn lettuce
Small box of raisins
½ cup cheese cubes
1 tomato cut in bite-size pieces
1 cup celery cut in bite-sizes
½ fresh lemon

Spoon yogurt into the bottom of a big bowl. Add dill and mix well. Now add all the other ingredients and toss until greens, etc. are coated with the yogurt-dill dressing. Top with a squeeze of fresh lemon.

Down on the Farm Salad

Another one for cottage cheese converts.

½ cup cottage cheese or ricotta, or ¼ cup of each
1 hard-boiled egg, chopped
¼ cucumber, sliced
½ tomato, in bite-size pieces
½ green pepper, in bite-size squares
¼ cup sunflower seeds
Cheddar cheese

Mix everything well and top with a mound of alfalfa sprouts and a dash of grated cheddar.

Banana Split au Naturel

Delicious and so very healthy.

Cottage cheese
1 large banana
½ cup granola
½ cup almonds
½ cup crushed strawberries

Use an ice cream scoop to put two mounds of cottage cheese on a plate. Slice the banana lengthwise and lay the halves flanking the cottage cheese scoops. Sprinkle with granola and almonds and top with crushed strawberries.

Nature's Favorite Salt Substitute
Float lemon slices in soup, or squeeze on vegetables, baked potatoes, salads, whatever. It's got the tang without the sodium.

Dinner: If you haven't had meat all day, then have it for dinner. *MAIN MEALS* Or have one of my "Main Meals" described below.

Bat Stew

Being a vegetarian I would never eat a bat, but mushrooms have that brown sweet little bat color.

1 large onion
½ pound thickly sliced mushrooms (you can cut them into bat shapes if you're really ambitious)
1 cup (½ pound) ricotta cheese
1 chopped tomato
1 cup baby green peas (fresh or frozen; canned peas have too much salt)

Put a small amount of vegetable oil in a saucepan and sauté onions and mushrooms until soft. Then add cheese, tomato, and green peas and stir until warmed through.

Shrimp Boat Special

What a way to end the day!

½ pound sliced mushrooms
1 cup cooked shrimp (canned OK)
3 tablespoons sherry
Brown rice

Put a small amount of vegetable oil in the saucepan and sauté mushrooms until soft. Add shrimp and sherry and stir until thoroughly warmed. Serve over prepared brown rice.

Eggplant Delight

Just as satisfying as meat.

2 large onions, chopped
1 cup diced celery
2 pounds eggplant (two medium) cut in ½-inch cubes
3 cups tomato sauce
Mozzarella cheese
Brown rice

Sauté onions and celery in a small amount of vegetable oil until clear. Add eggplant and tomato sauce and bring mixture to a boil. Then cover and let simmer for 45 minutes until the eggplant is very tender. Stir a bit from time to time. Serve over prepared brown rice and top with a thick slice of mozzarella cheese.

Potatoes Plus Punch

Either a side dish or a meal in itself.

1 onion, chopped
1 clove garlic, minced
8 ounces canned tomatoes, cut up
½ tablespoon basil
¼ tablespoon oregano
8 ounces grated sharp cheddar (2 cups)
1 ounce grated Parmesan (⅓ cup)
1 large baked potato

Sauté onion and garlic in a little vegetable oil until soft. Add tomatoes, basil, and oregano and bring to a simmer. Then add a handful at a time of the grated cheddar and Parmesan, stirring gently until each handful is melted before adding the next. Pour entire mixture over a hot split baked potato.

Charlie the Tuna

Serve it like an omelet.

3 eggs
1½ tablespoons milk
⅛ teaspoon dill
¾ ounces (half a small can) well-drained tuna (water-packed, please)
Grated mozzarella cheese

Mix the eggs, milk, and dill in a small bowl and scramble in a pan over low heat. As soon as the eggs begin to set, crumble in the tuna and sprinkle on the mozzarella. Remove pan from heat and cover until the cheese melts.

Green Bean Supreme

Direct from California.

3 cups cooked green beans
Cottage cheese, yogurt, *or* ricotta to taste
Alfalfa sprouts
Grated mozzarella
3 chopped raw carrots
1 cup sliced almonds

Mix cooked beans with cottage cheese, yogurt, or ricotta to taste. Top with alfalfa sprouts, grated mozzarella, raw carrots, and sliced onions in that order. If used alone as a main meal, serve with a slice of whole-wheat toast.

Dessert: To reward yourself for all those skipped candy bars and ice cream cones, have one of my "Dreamy Desserts." They're non-fattening (in moderation) and taste terrific!

Yogurt-on-a-Cloud

Virtue can be tasty.

2 cups plain yogurt
3 ounces frozen orange juice concentrate (½ a small can)
½ teaspoon vanilla
Ice cream sticks

Mix ingredients well in a blender and pour mixture into ice cube trays. Put in the freezer until semifrozen. Insert the ice cream sticks. Then let them freeze solid.

Banana-fanna Delight

4 medium ripe bananas
Carob sauce, maple syrup, *or* honey thinned with warm water
Chopped nuts *or* granola
Ice cream sticks

Peel the bananas, cut each in half, and trim about ⅛ inch off the tapered ends. Insert an ice cream stick in each, set the lot on a plate or pan, and freeze until firm. Then take the frozen bananas and either dip or roll each first in the syrup you've chosen, then roll in the nuts or granola. Eat right away, or put in an airtight container and return to the freezer.

Peanut Butter Log

¼ to ½ cup honey
½ cup peanut butter
2 cups (approx.) nonfat powdered milk

Knead ingredients until mixture holds together well. Then either roll into balls or shape into a log which can be cut in bite-size rounds. Chill well before serving.

Popcorn au Gratin

Too easy to be true.

Popcorn
Your favorite grated cheese

Pop a pot full of popcorn (easy on the oil, please). When popped, sprinkle with grated cheese and warm in a preheated 350-degree oven until cheese is melted. Let cool and dive in.

Strawberry Treat

½ cup ricotta cheese
1 cup fresh or frozen strawberries, slightly mashed
Granola
Sliced almonds
Shredded coconut

Spoon ricotta into a bowl and pour on the strawberries. (If berries were frozen be sure they're fully defrosted.) Mix gently and sprinkle with granola, almonds, and coconut to taste.

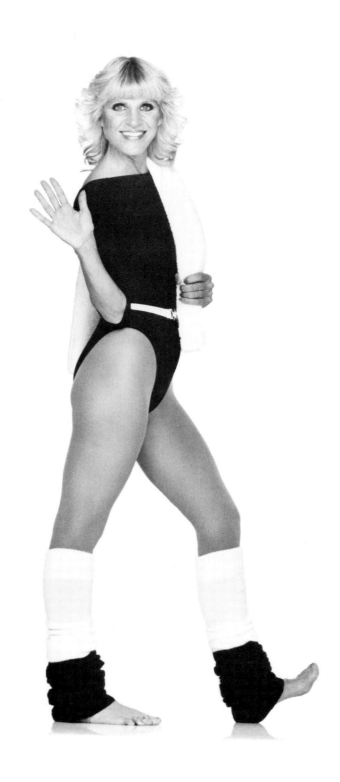

BYE-BYE!

Index

frequency of exercising and loss
of, 77
ideal weight range, 137
of muscle versus fat, 25
"set point," 138
uneven weight loss, 50
women's disadvantages in staying
slim, 99
Weights, hand-held, 37
Whole wheat products, 139
Wine, 140
Working heart rate, 3

Yogurt:
Green Bean Supreme, 148
-on-a-Cloud, 149
Saladorama, 144